O R M L

OXFORD RESPIRATORY MEDICINE LIBRARY

Chronic Obstructive Pulmonary Disease (COPD)

MAR 2011

CH

Oxford University Press makes no representation, express or implied, that the drug dosages in this book are correct. Readers must therefore always check the product information and clinical procedures with the most up-to-date published product information and data sheets provided by the manufacturers and the most recent codes of conduct and safety regulations. The authors and the publishers do not accept responsibility or legal liability for any errors in the text or for the misuse or misapplication of material in this work.

▶ Except where otherwise stated, drug doses and recommendations are for the non-pregnant adult who is not breast-feeding.

O R M L

OXFORD RESPIRATORY MEDICINE LIBRARY

Chronic Obstructive Pulmonary Disease (COPD)

Edited by

Dr Onn Min Kon

Imperial College Healthcare NHS Trust,
Chest and Allergy Clinic, St Mary's Hospital,
London, UK

Dr Trevor T. Hansel

National Heart & Lung Institute (NHLI),
Clinical Studies Unit, Imperial College,
London, UK

Professor Peter J. Barnes

Thoracic Medicine, National Heart and
Lung Institute (NHLI), Imperial College,
London, UK

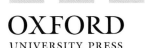

OXFORD
UNIVERSITY PRESS

OXFORD
UNIVERSITY PRESS

Great Clarendon Street, Oxford OX2 6DP

Oxford University Press is a department of the University of Oxford.
It furthers the University's objective of excellence in research, scholarship,
and education by publishing worldwide in

Oxford New York

Auckland Cape Town Dar es Salaam Hong Kong Karachi
Kuala Lumpur Madrid Melbourne Mexico City Nairobi
New Delhi Shanghai Taipei Toronto

With offices in

Argentina Austria Brazil Chile Czech Republic France Greece
Guatemala Hungary Italy Japan Poland Portugal Singapore
South Korea Switzerland Thailand Turkey Ukraine Vietnam

Oxford is a registered trade mark of Oxford University Press
in the UK and in certain other countries

Published in the United States
by Oxford University Press Inc., New York

British Library Cataloguing in Publication Data

Data available

Library of Congress Cataloging in Publication Data

Data available

Typeset by Newgen Imaging Systems (P) Ltd., Chennai, India
Printed in Great Britain
on acid-free paper by
Ashford Colour Press Ltd, Gosport, Hampshire

ISBN 978-0-19-954914-6

10 9 8 7 6 5 4 3 2 1

Contents

Contributors

Alvar GN Agustí
Servicio de Neumologia, Hospital Universitario Son Dureta Fundación Caubet-Cimera CIBR Enfermedades Respiratorias, Palma de Mallorca, Spain

Farid Bazari
Department of Respiratory Medicine, Royal Brompton Hospital, London, UK

Susannah A.A. Bloch
Imperial College Healthcare NHS Trust, St Mary's Hospital Chest and Allergy Clinic, London, UK

Aimee L. Brame
Chest and Allergy Clinic, St Mary's Hospital, Imperial College Healthcare NHS Trust, London, UK

Miguel Carrera
Servicio de Neumologia, Hospital Universitario Son Dureta Fundación Caubet-Cimera CIBER Enfermedades Respiratorias, Palma de Mallorca, Spain

Marc Decramer
Faculty of Kinesiology and Rehabilitation Sciences, Department of Rehabilitation Sciences, Katholieke Universiteit Leuven, Leuven, Belgium

Sarah L. Elkin
Chest and Allergy Clinic, St Mary's Hospital, Imperial College Healthcare NHS Trust, London, UK

Trevor T. Hansel
Medical Director, National Heart & Lung Institute (NHLI) Clinical Studies Unit, Imperial College School of Medicine, London, UK

David J. Jackson
Imperial College Healthcare NHS Trust, St Mary's Hospital Chest and Allergy Clinic, London, UK

Onn Min Kon
Chest and Allergy Clinic, St Mary's Hospital, Imperial College Healthcare NHS Trust, London, UK

Cassandra N.G. Lee
Chest and Allergy Clinic, St Mary's Hospital, Imperial College Healthcare NHS Trust, London, UK

William D. Man
National Institute of Health Research Clinician Scientist, Royal Brompton & Harefield NHS Trust, Kent, UK

CONTRIBUTORS

William L.G. Oldfield
Chest and Allergy Clinic,
St Mary's Hospital,
Imperial College Healthcare
NHS Trust, London, UK

Michael I. Polkey
Department of Respiratory
Medicine, Royal Brompton
Hospital, London, UK

Clare L.K. Ross
Imperial College Healthcare
NHS Trust, St Mary's
Hospital Chest and
Allergy Clinic,
London, UK

Ernest Sala
Servicio de Neumologia, Hospital
Universitario Son Dureta
Fundación Caubet-Cimera CIBER
Enfermedades Respiratorias,
Palma de Mallorca, Spain

Andrew J. Tan
National Heart and Lung
Institute (NHLI) Clinical
Studies Unit, Imperial College
School of Medicine, London, UK

Thierry Troosters
Respiratory Rehabilitation
and Respiratory Division,
University Hospital, Leuven
Leuven, Belgium

Abbreviations

α1-PI	α1–Protease inhibitor
6MWD	six-minute walking distance
6MWT	six-minute walk test
ABG	arterial blood gas
AHR	airway hyperresponsiveness
ALK-5	activin-like receptor kinase
AO	ambulatory oxygen
ATS	American Thoracic Society
BAL	bronchoalveolar lavage
BDR	bronchodilator reversibility
BMI	body mass index
CO	carbon monoxide
COPD	chronic obstructive pulmonary disease
CTGF	connective tissue growth factor
CPAP	continuous positive airway pressure
CPET	cardio-pulmonary exercise testing
CPR	cardiopulmonary resuscitation
CRDQ-Dys	dyspnea subscale of the chronic respiratory disease questionnaire
CXR	chest X-ray
cAMP	cyclic adenosine monophosphate
CCR2	cysteine–cysteine receptor 2
CT	computed tomography
CXCR2	cysteine-X-cysteine receptor 2
DH	dynamic hyperinflation
DLCO	diffusing capacity for carbon monoxide
DPI	dry powder inhalers
ET-1	endothelin-1
EPHX	epoxide hydrolase
EGF	epidermal growth factor
ERV	expiratory reserve volume
EPAP	expiratory positive airway pressure
ECM	extracellular matrix
FEV1	forced expiratory volume in one second
FFM	fat-free mass
FRC	functional residual capacity
FVC	forced vital capacity
GOLD	Global Initiative for Chronic Obstructive Lung Disease
GRO-α	growth-related oncogene
GSTM1	glutathione-S-transferase M1

GWA	genome-wide linkage analysis
HRCT	high-resolution computerized tomography
HIV	human immunodeficiency virus
HMOX	heme oxygenase
HaH	Hospital-at-Home
HU	Hounsfield unit
HRQoL	Health-related Quality of Life
HOCl	hypochlorous acid
ICS	inhaled corticosteroids
IFN-γ	interferon-γ
IL-13	interleukin-13
IPAP	inspiratory positive airway pressure
IPF	idiopathic pulmonary fibrosis
IMV	invasive mechanical ventilation
IRV	inspiratory reserve volume
JVP	jugular venous pressure
LTB4	leukotriene B4
LHS	Lung Health Study
LPS	lipopolysaccharide
LLN	lower limit of normal
LTOT	long-term oxygen therapy
LABA	long-acting β_2-agonist
LAMA	long-acting muscarinic antagonist
LVRS	lung volume reduction surgery
MR	magnetic resonance
MMPs	matrix metalloproteases
MRC	Medical Research Council
MDI	metered dose inhalers
MCP-1	monocyte chemotactic peptide-1
NETT	National Emphysema Treatment Trial
NMES	neuromuscular electrical stimulation
NE	neutrophil elastase
NADPH	nicotinamide adenine dinucleotide phosphate
nACh	nicotinic acetylcholine receptors
NOS	nitric oxide synthase
NIPPV	non-invasive positive pressure ventilation
NIV	non-invasive ventilation
PEF	peak of expiratory curve
PDGF	platelet-derived growth factor
PEEP	positive-end expiratory pressure
PAR-2	protease activated receptor 2
RNS	reactive nitrogen species

ROS	reactive oxidant species
RV	residual volume
RBILD	respiratory bronchiolitis-associated interstitial lung disease
RR	respiratory rate
SLPI	secretory leukocyte protease inhibitor
SERPIN	serine protease inhibitor
SFTPB	surfactant protein B
SGRQ	Saint George's Respiratory Questionnaire
SBOT	short-burst oxygen therapy
SABA	short-acting β_2-agonist
SOB	shortness of breath
SOD	superoxide dismutase
SCM	sternocleidomastoid
TIMPs	tissue inhibitors of metalloproteinases
TLRs	toll-like receptors
TLC	total lung capacity
TLCO	transfer factor of the lung for carbon monoxide
TGF-β	transforming growth factor-β_1
TNFα	tumour necrosis factor α
TV	tidal volume
VEGF	vascular endothelial growth factor
VC	vital capacity
VAT	video-assisted thoracoscopy

Chapter 1

Global burden and natural history of COPD

Trevor T. Hansel and Onn Min Kon

Key points

- The Global Initiative for Chronic Obstructive Lung Disease (GOLD, 2007) defines COPD as a non-reversible, progressive, obstructive lung disease generally caused by the inhalation of noxious gases and particles. COPD is recognized as being both preventable and treatable.
- The diagnosis of COPD is frequently made at a late stage, as many patients ignore early symptoms of cough and exertional dyspnea.
- The severity of COPD is commonly assessed by spirometry, in terms of the post-bronchodilator forced expiratory volume in one second (FEV_1).
- COPD is generally caused by tobacco smoking, but it is also caused by inhalation of smoke from burning biomass fuel in developing countries.
- Tobacco smoking is rising globally because of increased smoking in many low-income countries.
- In 2001 COPD was the fifth leading cause of death in high-income countries and the sixth leading cause of death in nations of low and middle income.
- A series of genes have been associated with COPD and emphysema, but many of these associations have not been confirmed.
- The annual rate of decline in FEV_1 is the classical measure of the natural history of COPD.
- Extrapulmonary systemic features of COPD include muscle weakness and wasting, cachexia, cardiovascular disease, metabolic syndrome, endocrine defects, anaemia, depression, and malignancies.

1.1 Definition of COPD

1.1.1 GOLD 2007 definition

The GOLD 2007 working definition of COPD recognizes the importance of 'noxious particles or gases' in causing the airflow limitation of COPD, when cigarette smoking is the major cause in 95% of cases in industrialized societies (Table 1.1). COPD may also be caused by exposure to mineral dusts, fumes from indoor biomass fuels, and outdoor air pollution. These latter risk factors are of more significance in developing rather than developed countries. The obstructive lung defect typical of COPD comprises a decreased FEV_1 compared to that predicted for an individual. The FEV_1 should be measured following inhalation of a bronchodilator and expressed as a percentage of that predicted for the individual. COPD was formerly considered to be defined by non-reversible or fixed airflow limitation (Figure 1.1). Reversibility has been found to be a continuous variable in COPD patients, does not predict disease progression, and varies between visits.

Table 1.1 Differential diagnosis of COPD	
Disease	Suggestive features
COPD	Onset in middle age and elderly
	History of tobacco smoking
	Slowly progressive symptoms: shortness of breath (SOB) on exertion
Asthma	Onset in childhood
	Variable symptoms: episodic SOB with wheeze
	Trigger factors: infection, allergens, exercise, emotion
	History of allergy, sputum eosinophilia
	Reversible to bronchodilators, responds to inhaled corticosteroids (ICS)
Congestive heart failure	Basal crackles: pulmonary and ankle oedema
	Cardiomegaly on Chest X-ray
Bronchiectasis	Large volume purulent sputum
	CXR: bronchial dilation and thickening
Tuberculosis	CXR is often helpful
	Endemic areas, vulnerable populations
	Microbiological confirmation

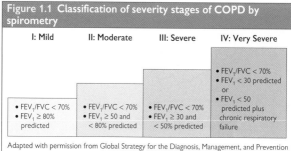

Figure 1.1 Classification of severity stages of COPD by spirometry

I: Mild	II: Moderate	III: Severe	IV: Very Severe
• FEV$_1$/FVC < 70% • FEV$_1$ ≥ 80% predicted	• FEV$_1$/FVC < 70% • FEV$_1$ ≥ 50 and < 80% predicted	• FEV$_1$/FVC < 70% • FEV$_1$ ≥ 30 and < 50% predicted	• FEV$_1$/FVC < 70% • FEV$_1$ < 30 predicted or • FEV$_1$ < 50 predicted plus chronic respiratory failure

Adapted with permission from Global Strategy for the Diagnosis, Management, and Prevention of Chronic Obstructive Pulmonary Disease (Updated in 2007). © Gold, www.goldcopd.com

1.1.2 Spirometric classification of the severity of COPD (GOLD 2007)

According to the GOLD guidelines of 2007, post-bronchodilator FEV$_1$ is recommended for the diagnosis and assessment of severity of COPD (Figure 1.1), and on this basis there are four stages in the classification of the severity of COPD. Use of the lower limit of normal (LLN) of the post-bronchodilator FEV$_1$/forced vital capacity ratio should be used to confirm irreversible airflow obstruction.

1.2 The burden of COPD

- The WHO Global Burden of Disease Project estimated that COPD was the sixth leading cause of death in 1990 and that it will become the third leading cause of death by 2020
- Prevalence data for COPD is derived mostly from industrial countries; however, there is a consensus that there has been a worldwide increase in COPD due to increases in cigarette smoking in developing countries
- Tobacco smoking rates are 49% for men and 8% for women in low- and middle-income countries, and 37% for men and 21% for women in high-income countries
- Figures are generally greatly underestimated because COPD is frequently not diagnosed until it is clinically apparent and moderately advanced, and death from COPD may be due to secondary complications such as heart failure
- There were approximately 2.7 million deaths from COPD in 2000, half of them occurring in the Western Pacific Region, with most taking place in China. About 400,000 deaths occur each year from COPD in industrialized societies

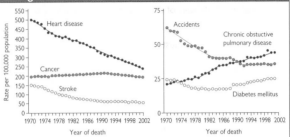

Figure 1.2 Trends in age-standardized death rates for the six leading causes of death

Reference: Jemal A, Ward E, Hao YP, and Thun M (2005). Trends in the leading causes of death in the United States, 1970–2002. *JAMA*, **294**, 1255–9.

- In a systematic review and meta-analysis, the pooled prevalence of COPD was 7.6% from 37 studies, with the pooled prevalence from 26 spirometric studies being 8.9%
- In a study of age-standardized death rates from all causes in the United States, among the six leading causes of death, COPD deaths doubled from 1970 to 2002 (Figure 1.2).

1.3 Environmental causes of COPD

1.3.1 Tobacco smoking

Cigarette smoking is by far the commonest cause of COPD worldwide, accounting for more than 95% of cases in industrialized countries, but it should not be forgotten that some patients with COPD are non-smokers. Usually there is a smoking history of greater than 20 pack-years. Pipe and cigar smokers have a higher risk of COPD than non-smokers, although rates are lower than those for cigarette smokers. Passive smoking is associated with COPD possibly via effects on lung growth during childhood. Smoking during pregnancy may also be a risk factor for COPD as this may affect foetal lung growth.

1.3.2 Air pollution: outdoor and indoor

Air pollution, particularly sulphur dioxide and particulates (black smoke or particulate matter of ≤10 μm [PM_{10}]), is associated with chronic simple bronchitis and COPD. There may be interactions between cigarette smoking and air pollution. In places where there is heavy air pollution, this may be as important a risk factor as cigarette smoking. Indoor air pollution from biomass fuel that is burned for cooking and heating in poorly ventilated homes may be an important risk factor for COPD in developing countries and this may account for the relatively high rates of disease amongst women.

1.3.3 Occupational exposure: inorganic and organic

Occupational exposure to dusts (coal, silica, quartz), isocyanate fumes, and solvents may be significant. These noxious agents may interact with cigarette smoke to cause COPD. The importance of occupational dust exposure to coal and gold miners is probably underestimated. Exposure to cadmium, welding fumes, and organic dusts may also be associated with emphysema.

1.3.4 Respiratory infections

Both viral and bacterial chest infections during the first year of life are associated with COPD in later life, and infections in childhood may play a role. There is also evidence that certain latent virus infections (such as adenovirus) may cause amplification of inflammation in emphysema and predispose to the development of COPD. Human immunodeficiency virus (HIV) seropositive smokers have increased susceptibility to emphysema. The Lung Health Study (LHS) has noted that lower respiratory illnesses promote FEV_1 decline in current smokers, and exacerbation frequency also contributes to the rate of lung function decline.

1.3.5 Atopy, airway hyperresponsiveness (AHR), and asthma

There has been considerable debate about the influence of atopy and AHR on the development of COPD. The 'Dutch hypothesis' proposed that atopy and IgE underlie the development of COPD. This hypothesis claims that asthma and COPD are two extremes of the same basic process, while GOLD stresses the differences between the clinical features, pathology, and pharmacology of these diseases. COPD itself may result in increased airway responsiveness to histamine or methacholine owing to geometric factors related to fixed airway narrowing. Nevertheless, there is increased bronchodilator responsiveness among first-degree currently smoking and ex-smoking relatives of patients with early-onset COPD. Airways responsiveness is associated with the development of chronic respiratory symptoms, mortality from COPD increases with more severe AHR to histamine, and bronchodilator reversibility is associated with increased survival in COPD patients. Adults with asthma have been found to have a higher risk of acquiring COPD with time than those without asthma, after adjusting for smoking.

1.3.6 **Dietary factors and oxidative stress**

- Low dietary intake of antioxidant vitamins (A, C, and E)
- Beneficial effects have been described for fish oil and flavonoids (especially catechins) in solid fruits and vegetables
- Alcohol consumption has been found to be protective in heavy smokers.

1.3.7 **Nutrition and lung growth and development**

Early nutrition may be important, and small-for-dates babies have an increased risk of development of COPD in later life. Patients with emphysema are more likely to have a low birth weight and be underweight in adult life, while those with chronic bronchitis are more likely to be obese. Cachexia with dramatic weight loss can itself be part of the clinical features of severe COPD.

1.3.8 **Gender and socioeconomic status**

It is controversial whether females are more susceptible than men to the effects of cigarette smoking, although a range of studies have found greater prevalence of COPD in women. In developing countries women may have greater exposure to air pollution from burning cooking fuels. There is evidence that the risk of developing COPD is inversely related to socioeconomic status.

1.4 **Genetics of COPD**

- The archetypical gene for early-onset COPD is the ZZ allele (piZ phenotype) of the α_1-protease inhibitor gene (α_1-PI, α_1-antitrypsin), but it accounts for less than 1% of cases of COPD in Northern Europe. α_1-PI is a serine protease inhibitor (SERPIN) which primarily combats neutrophil elastase.
- COPD is a polygenic disease, but there has been failure to replicate many of the initial gene association studies on COPD and emphysema (see Table 1.2, and review by Hersh and colleagues, 2008), and this is partly because of issues in phenotype definition.
- Recently, genome wide linkage analysis (GWA) has led to identification of two promising candidate genes for COPD: TGFβ1 and SERPINE2.
- Candidate genes include proteases and their inhibitors, xenobiotic metabolizing enzymes, immune system modulators, and genes for addictive behaviour.

Table 1.2 Candidate genes associated with COPD and emphysema
Genes
Proteases and inhibitors   • α_1 antitrypsin (AAT = SERPINA1)   • SERPINE2   • α_1 antichymotrypsin (SERPINA3)   • Matrix metallopeptidase-9 (MMP-9)
Xenobiotic metabolizing enzymes: • Microsomal epoxide hydrolase (EPHX1)   • Glutathione-S-transferase M1 (GSTM1)   • Extracellular superoxide dismutase (SOD3)   • Heme oxygenase (HMOX1)
Cytokines: TGF-β1   TNF-α
Surfactant protein B (SFTPB)
Addictive behaviour: SLC6A3 dopamine transporter and DRD2 dopamine receptor.

1.5 Natural history of COPD

1.5.1 Spirometry

The classic British study of Fletcher and Peto undertaken in 792 London working men aged 30–59 years over an eight-year period demonstrated that the hallmark of COPD is an accelerated rate of decline of FEV_1 (Figure 1.3). From this time, the measurement of the rate of loss of FEV_1 on an annual basis is the classical means of recording the natural history of COPD.

The North American Lung Health Study was a clinical trial involving smoking cessation in 5,887 middle-aged smokers with mild-to-moderate COPD with FEV_1 at 50–90% predicted (Figure 1.3). There was a slight improvement in FEV_1 over the first year after cessation, depending on the severity of the COPD, followed by a slower rate of decline in sustained quitters compared to continuing smokers over 5 years, which was confirmed at 11 years. Interestingly, smokers who give up cigarettes when they have higher FEV_1 recordings have greater benefit from smoking cessation, and patients with more severe COPD show less benefit in terms of FEV_1 a year after cessation.

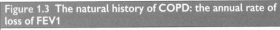

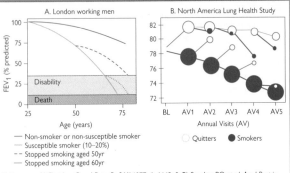

Figure 1.3 The natural history of COPD: the annual rate of loss of FEV1

A. London working men

B. North America Lung Health Study

— Non-smoker or non-susceptible smoker
— Susceptible smoker (10–20%)
-- Stopped smoking aged 50yr
— Stopped smoking aged 60yr

○ Quitters   ● Smokers

References: A) Fletcher C and Peto R. *BMJ* 1977; **1**: 1645–8; B) Scanlon PO *et al. Am J Respir Crit Care Med* 2000; **161**: 381–90, © American Thoracic Society.

1.5.2 The BODE index and systemic COPD

In more severe COPD it is important to also assess systemic features of COPD; hence the BODE index is a useful predictor of mortality:

- **B**MI: body mass index or fat-free mass (FFM)
- **O**bstruction: FEV$_1$ on spirometry
- **D**yspnoea score
- **E**xercise performance: six-minute walk test (6MWT).

Key reference

National Institutes of Health (NIH), National Heart Lung and Blood Institute (NHLBI), World Health Organization (WHO). *Global Initiative for Chronic Obstructive Lung Disease (GOLD): Global Strategy for the Diagnosis, Management, and Prevention of Chronic Obstructive Pulmonary Disease.* Updated 2007.

References

Celli BR and Barnes PJ (2007). Exacerbations of chronic obstructive pulmonary disease. *Eur Respir J,* **29**(6), 1224–38.

Celli BR, Cote CG, and Marin JM *et al.* (2004). The body-mass index, airflow obstruction, dyspnea, and exercise capacity index in chronic obstructive pulmonary disease. *N Engl J Med,* **350**(10), 1005–12.

Cookson WOC (2008). Genetics and genomics of chronic obstructive pulmonary disease. *Proc Am Thorac oc,* **3**, 473–7.

Halbert RJ, Natoli JL, Gano A, Badamgarav E, Buist AS, and Mannino DM (2006). Global burden of COPD: systematic review and meta-analysis. *Eur Respir J,* **28**(3), 523–32.

Hersh CP, DeMeo DL, and Silverman EK (2008). National emphysema treatment trial state of the art: genetics of emphysema. *Proc Am Thorac Soc*, **5**(4), 486–93.

Jemal A, Ward E, Hao YP, and Thun M (2005). Trends in the leading causes of death in the United States, 1970–2002. *JAMA*, **294**, 1255–9.

Lopez AD, Shibuya K, and Rao C *et al.* (2006). Chronic obstructive pulmonary disease: current burden and future projections. *Eur Respir J*, **27**(2), 397–412.

Mannino DM and Buist AS (2007). Global burden of COPD: risk factors, prevalence, and future trends. *Lancet*, **370**(9589), 765–73.

Mannino DM, Watt G, and Hole D *et al.* (2006). The natural history of chronic obstructive pulmonary disease. *Eur Respir J*, **27**(3), 627–43.

Yanbaeva DG, Dentener MA, Creutzberg EC, Wesseling G, and Wouters EF (2007). Systemic effects of smoking. *Chest*, **131**(5), 1557–66.

Chapter 2

Pathology and molecular features of COPD

Trevor T. Hansel, Andrew J. Tan, and Onn Min Kon

Key points

- Cigarette smoke is estimated to contain 1017 reactive oxidant species (ROS) and chronic smoking in genetically susceptible individuals is the major environmental risk factor for chronic obstructive pulmonary disease (COPD).
- COPD involves a spectrum of diseases: chronic bronchitis, obstructive bronchiolitis, emphysema, pulmonary vascular disease, *cor pulmonale*, and a systemic syndrome of cachexia and muscle weakness.
- ROS trigger an exaggerated host inflammatory, mucosecretory, proteolytic, and fibrotic response. Epithelial cell injury and macrophage activation causes release of chemotactic factors and cytokines such as CXCL1, CXCL8, CCL2, and TNF-α.
- Macrophages and neutrophils then release proteases, with involvement of matrix metalloproteases (MMPs) and neutrophil elastase (NE) that may break down extracellular matrix (ECM). T cells of various subtypes (Th1, Th2, Tc1, Tc2, Treg, Th17) as well as B cells may also be involved in this inflammatory cascade.
- Transforming growth factor-β1 (TGF-β1) is produced by epithelial cells and causes fibrosis. Inhibition of fibrosis is caused by interferon-γ (IFN-γ), while profibrotic factors include interleukin-13 (IL-13), platelet-derived growth factor (PDGF), CCL2 (MCP-1) and CXCL12 (ligand for CXCR4), and protease activated receptor 2 (PAR-2).
- Many years of injury from cigarette smoke causes cycles of inflammation and repair. These cycles may result in resolution, but are commonly associated with mucus hypersecretion, fibrosis, proteolysis, and both airway and parenchymal remodelling.

2.1 **The modern definition of COPD**

The Global Initiative for Chronic Obstructive Lung Disease (GOLD) has recently formulated a working definition of COPD that reflects that airflow limitation is usually associated with an abnormal inflammatory response of the lung to noxious particles or gases.

2.2 **The pathology of COPD**

At five separate anatomical sites different pathological events occur, with distinct physiological sequelae, that result in varying clinical manifestations: chronic bronchitis, obstructive bronchiolitis, emphysema, pulmonary vascular disease and *cor pulmonale*, systemic disease with cachexia, and respiratory and peripheral muscle weakness. In the large airways there is chronic bronchitis and increased mucus secretion, in the small airways there is fibrosis and obstructive bronchiolitis, while in the lung interstitium there is parenchymal damage and emphysema (Figure 2.1).

2.2.1 **Chronic bronchitis**

Chronic (simple) bronchitis is defined clinically by a productive cough on most days for at least three months for at least two consecutive years that cannot be attributed to other pulmonary or cardiac causes (Medical Research Council [MRC]). Chronic bronchitis is a consequence of mucus hyperplasia, resulting in hypersecretion of mucus, and the term 'chronic bronchitis' can also be used to describe histopathological features. Patients with established airway obstruction and associated mucus hypersecretion have a worst prognosis. However, a 15-year study has found that chronic bronchitis does not have increased risk of subsequent airways obstruction.

2.2.2 **Obstructive bronchiolitis**

Obstructive bronchiolitis is due to obstruction of peripheral airways as a result of an inflammatory response, with a type of fibrosis involving airway remodelling. Airway remodelling, loss of alveolar attachments, and excess mucus are all believed to contribute to obstruction and collapse of small airways. Obstructive bronchiolitis involves the small or peripheral airways, and is an inflammatory condition of small airways less than 2mm in internal diameter (Figure 2.1). Histologically, an early effect of cigarette smoke in patients with COPD is a marked increase in the number of macrophages, neutrophil, and CD8+ T cells in the bronchioli, and an associated respiratory bronchiolitis and alveolitis. The important study of Hogg and colleagues demonstrated that progression of COPD is associated with inflammation, small airway thickening and fibrosis, and mucous exudates. In severe COPD lymphoid follicles were noted around small airways.

Figure 2.1 Pathology of COPD

Chronic bronchitis

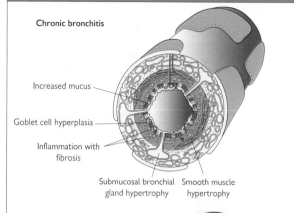

Increased mucus

Goblet cell hyperplasia

Inflammation with
fibrosis

Submucosal bronchial   Smooth muscle
gland hypertrophy   hypertrophy

Obstructive bronchiolitis

Collapsed lumen

Increased mucus

Goblet cells metaplasia

Smooth muscle
hypertrophy

Loss of alveolar
attachments

Inflammation with fibrosis

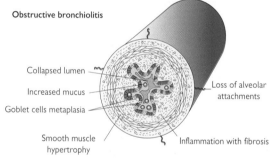

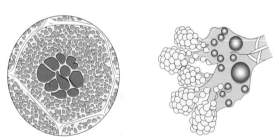

Chronic bronchitis is characterized by increased mucus production, globlet cell hyperplasia, and
submucosal hypertrophy. In obstructive bronchiolitis, collapse of the lumen and fibrosis of the
thickened and inflamed wall are prominent. Centrilobular emphysema consists of destructive
enlargement and confluence of the third-order respiratory bronchioles. Centrilobular emphysema
predominantly affects the upper lobes.

2.2.3 **Emphysema**

Emphysema is a pathological diagnosis characterized by destruction of alveolar walls, resulting in abnormal and permanent enlargement (dilatation) of airspaces and loss of lung elasticity, with consequent obstruction of peripheral airways. Emphysema is defined by permanent, destructive enlargement of the airspaces distal to the terminal bronchioli, affecting the respiratory bronchioles and the alveoli (Figure 2.1). The mechanism of this process is poorly understood, but it is thought to be an inflammatory condition of the lung parenchyma mediated by T-lymphocytes, neutrophils, and alveolar macrophages; the latter cells causing the release of excessive amounts of proteolytic enzymes such as NE and MMPs. Inflammation and proteolysis are accompanied by destruction of lung parenchyma, fibrosis, and remodelling.

Centrilobular emphysema is the most common cause of cigarette smoking induced emphysema in COPD. It involves the dilatation and destruction of the respiratory bronchioles. Centrilobular emphysema occurs more frequently in the upper lung fields in mild disease. In more advanced disease, lesions are more diffuse and also involve destruction of the capillary bed. Later changes involve the loss of the interacinar septa, as well as the airspace walls. This may lead to progressively enlarging holes, >1mm in diameter, which can be visualized on high-resolution computerized tomography (HRCT). The destructive process of emphysema is accompanied by a net increase in the mass of collagen with alveolar wall fibrosis.

2.2.4 **Pulmonary vascular disease**

Pulmonary vascular disease begins early in the course of COPD as intimal thickening, followed by smooth muscle hypertrophy and inflammatory infiltration. This may be followed by pulmonary hypertension and destruction of the capillary bed. Endothelin-1 (ET-1) is strongly expressed in pulmonary vascular endothelium of patients with pulmonary hypertension secondary to chronic hypoxia. Although pulmonary hypertension and *cor pulmonale* are common sequelae of COPD, the precise mechanisms of increased vascular resistance are unclear.

2.2.5 **Systemic COPD**

Systemic features of COPD include disturbances in metabolism with cachexia, as well as increased respiratory and skeletal muscle fatigue with wasting. Patients with predominant emphysema may develop profound weight loss, and this is a predictor of increased mortality. The BODE score of BMI, obstruction of airways, dyspnoea, and reduced exercise capacity is predictive of mortality. Weight loss in COPD has been associated with increased levels of tumour necrosis factor α (TNFα) and soluble TNFα receptors. The skeletal muscle weakness may exacerbate dyspnoea, and skeletal and respiratory muscle training is an important aspect of pulmonary rehabilitation. The metabolic syndrome, male hypogonadism, thyroid disorders, anaemia, depression, cardiovascular disease, and a range of malignancies are associated with COPD.

2.3 Cellular involvement

Cigarette smoke and other inhaled irritants initiate an inflammatory response in the peripheral airways and lung parenchyma (Figure 2.2). Over many years of injury, cycles of inflammation and repair occur that may result in resolution, but can be associated with excess mucus production, proteolysis, fibrosis, and both airway and parenchymal remodelling. Inflammation in 'healthy' smokers is very similar to that in COPD, in terms of inflammatory cells, mediators, and proteases, but is less pronounced. This suggests that the inflammation in COPD represents an exaggeration of the normal inflammatory response to noxious agents.

2.3.1 Macrophages

Macrophages are activated by cigarette smoke and other inhaled irritants, and macrophage numbers are increased in bronchoalveolar lavage (BAL) fluid of patients with COPD, and are concentrated in the centriacinar zones where emphysema is most marked. Alveolar macrophages are long-lived cells, and there is indirect evidence that they may have prolonged survival in COPD, since the anti-apoptotic protein Bcl-XL is increased. Significant increases are reported in the numbers of subepithelial CD68+ macrophages in chronic bronchitis.

2.3.2 Neutrophils

It is not understood why the increased number of neutrophils found in BAL fluid and sputum from subjects with COPD is not usually seen in the bronchial mucosa, at least in the subepithelial zone where the biopsy is generally quantified. This may be due to rapid transit of neutrophils through the airways and parenchyma. Interestingly, rapid decline in FEV_1 in smokers is associated with increased levels of sputum neutrophils. Toll-like receptors (TLRs) respond to oxidants, bacterial lipopolysaccharide (LPS), and viral motifs and are important in generating neutrophilic inflammation.

2.3.3 T-lymphocytes

Increased numbers of various T-cell populations have been variously described in COPD : Tc1, Tc2, Th1, Th2, Th17 and Tregs. In COPD the CD8+ (cytotoxic/suppressor) lymphocyte increases in number

Figure 2.2 Radical pathways from cigarette smoke and in COPD airways

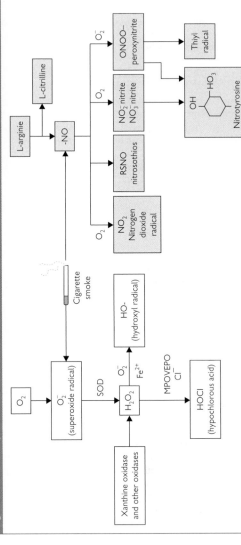

Oxygen is converted to superoxide radical by the action of oxidases, and through interaction with semiquinone radicals in the tar phase of cigarette smoke. Superoxide is then metabolized to hydrogen peroxide, hydroxyl radical, and hypochlorous acid (HOCl). Nitric oxide, itself a free radical, is present in the gas phase of cigarette smoke and is also produced by the action of nitric oxide synthase (NOS). Nitric oxide is metabolized to a range of nitrogen-containing radicals, nitrosothiols, and nitrotyrosine.

and proportion to become the predominant T-cell subset. Th17 cells are especially important in neutrophilic responses. The increase of the CD8 phenotype and of the CD8/CD4 ratio occurs in both the mucosa and submucosa, and is associated with increased mucus-secreting glands. These cells may contribute to pathophysiology via the release of granzymes, perforins, and TNFα that induce apoptosis in type I alveolar cells. In stable mild/moderate COPD there is Tc1 activation with production of IFN-γ. Lymphocyte distribution is suggestive of reactive changes in the lymphoid follicles associated with small airways of more severe COPD.

2.3.4 Eosinophils

There are some reports of increased numbers of inactive eosinophils in the airways and BAL of patients with stable COPD, although others have not found these increases. It has been noted that the presence of eosinophils predicts a response to corticosteroids and may indicate coexisting asthma with COPD. Airways resected from the lungs of heavy smokers demonstrate marked gene expression for both IL-4 and IL-5, and this eosinophilia is associated with the bronchial glands of subjects with chronic bronchitis. However, the most pronounced eosinophilia occurs when there is an exacerbation of COPD.

2.3.5 Epithelial cells

Airway epithelial cells are likely to be an important source of mediators in COPD. Epithelial cells are activated by cigarette smoke to produce TNFα and CXCL8, while TGF-β may induce local fibrosis. However, it has also be shown that cigarette smoke extract can inhibit CXCL8 mRNA expression and expression of cytokines. Vascular endothelial growth factor (VEGF) may be necessary to maintain alveolar cell survival.

2.4 Molecular features

2.4.1 Reactive oxidative species (ROS)

Both the gas phase of cigarette smoke and the tar component can lead to the generation of ROS (Figure 2.3). In addition to direct inhalation of ROS from cigarette smoke, the inflammatory processes that occur in smoker's lungs can lead to further generation of oxidants by nicotinamide adenine dinucleotide phosphate (NADPH) oxidase in leukocytes drawn to the site of inflammation. ROS include superoxide anion (O_2^-), hydrogen peroxide (H_2O_2) and hydroxyl radicals (.OH). O_2^- may be converted to H_2O_2 by superoxide dismutase (SOD).

Reactive nitrogen species (RNS) includes nitric oxide (.NO) and its derivatives such as nitrogen dioxide (NO_2) and peroxynitrite ($ONOO^-$) (Figure 2.3). Nitric oxide (.NO) is itself a gaseous radical

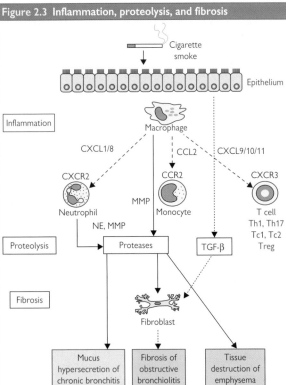

Figure 2.3 Inflammation, proteolysis, and fibrosis

Oxidants within cigarette smoke, as well as other irritants, activate epithelial cells and macrophages in the respiratory tract which release neutrophil chemotactic factors, including CXCL8 (IL-8) and leukotriene B4 (LTB4). The IL-8 family causes chemotaxis of neutrophils via the cysteine-X-cysteine receptor 2 (CXCR2), while CCL2 (monocyte chemotactic peptide-1, MCP-1) binds to cysteine–cysteine receptor 2 (CCR2). Cytotoxic CD8+ T cells may also be involved in the inflammatory cascade. Neutrophils and tissue macrophages are a potent source of oxidants (O_2^-) and proteases, the latter being normally inhibited by a panel of endogenous protease inhibitors. Proteases include NE, cathepsins, and various MMPs. Fibroblasts are a prominent feature in the pathology of bronchiolitis and emphysema, and regenerative healing processes, as well as tissue remodelling, occur in COPD. TGF-β is a potent stimulator of collagen production by fibroblasts.

Reactive nitrogen species (RNS) includes nitric oxide (.NO) and its derivatives such as nitrogen dioxide (NO_2) and peroxynitrite ($ONOO^-$) (Figure 2.3). Nitric oxide (.NO) is itself a gaseous radical and has complex regulatory actions in a variety of inflammatory and infectious conditions. Nitric oxide synthase (NOS) converts L-arginine to L-citrulline and generates .NO. O_2^- can react with .NO to form ONOO⁻, a very unstable and highly reactive molecule that mediates many of the damaging effects of oxidative stress. Nitrite (NO_2^-) is a major end product of .NO metabolism that is rapidly metabolized to nitrate (NO_3^-) and has been shown to promote tyrosine nitration by reaction with HOCl. Myeloperoxidase has the capacity to produce nitrating oxidants and may also produce nitrate tyrosine residues. Oxidants have the capacity to stimulate inflammation through TLR.

2.4.2 Epidermal growth factor (EGF)

Mucus hypersecretion may arise through activation of sensory nerve endings in the airways through reflex (local peptidergic and spinal cholinergic) pathways and direct stimulatory effects of enzymes such as NE. Recent studies suggest that EGF is a key mediator of mucus hyperplasia and mucus hypersecretion. Chronic stimulation leads to upregulation of mucin (MUC) genes, especially MUC5B in the bronchiolar lumen and MUC5AC in the bronchiolar epithelium.

2.4.3 Chemoattractants, cytokines, and chemokines

CXCR1/CXCR2: CXCL8 (IL-8) is secreted by macrophages, neutrophils, and by airway epithelial cells and binds to the receptors CXCR1 and CXCR2. The low-affinity CXCR1 is specific for CXCL8 and is involved in neutrophil activation. The high-affinity CXCR2 is activated by a range of CXC chemokines including CXCL8 and CXCL1 (growth-related oncogene, GRO-α), and is involved in the chemotaxis of neutrophils and monocytes. There are increased amounts of neutrophils, LTB4, and CXCL8 in induced sputum of patients with COPD, and chemokine receptors are important therapeutic targets in COPD.

CCR2: In addition, CCL2 (macrophage chemotactic peptide-1, MCP-1) is a potent chemoattractant for monocytes, which acts via CCR2. There are increased numbers of macrophages in the interstitium that are derived from blood monocytes in COPD.

CXCL9, CXCL10, and CXC11: These are chemotactic for various T-cell populations.

TNFα: This is present in high concentration in the sputum of COPD patients, especially during exacerbations. TNFα may activate the transcription of NF-κB, which switches on the transcription of inflammatory genes, including chemokine genes and proteases, in macrophages and epithelial cells.

2.4.4 Protease–antiprotease balance

The key to the pathogenesis of emphysema is believed to be an imbalance of proteases and antiproteases in the lung. Neutrophils and macrophages together secrete proteases capable of digesting all the components of the ECM in the lung interstitium. Emphysema is characterised by a loss of elastic recoil, with destruction of components of the ECM including elastin fibres. The ECM is a dynamic structure, which requires equilibrium between the synthesis and degradation of its components to maintain homeostasis. Proteases are also potent stimulators of mucus secretion.

- Serine proteases (NE, cathepsin G, and protease 3) and cysteine proteases (cathepsins) are produced by neutrophils
- MMPs are a group of more than 20 closely related endopeptidases produced by both neutrophils and alveolar macrophages as well as airway epithelial cells. MMPs have various substrate specificities: collagenase (MMPs-1 and 8) and elastolysis through MMP-2 (gelatinase A), MMP-9, and MMP-12 (macrophage metalloelastase)
- α_1–Protease inhibitor (α_1-PI, α_1-antitrypsin) is the main inhibitor of NE, and individuals with a congenital deficiency of α_1-PI are susceptible to the early development of emphysema
- α_1-Anti-chymotrypsin
- Secretory leukocyte protease inhibitor (SLPI)
- Tissue inhibitors of metalloproteinases (TIMPs) counteract the effect of MMPs. MMP-9/TIMP-1 ratios correlate with FEV_1, suggesting that there is a protease/antiprotease imbalance in favour of fibrosis in patients with airway obstruction but not emphysema.

2.4.5 Fibrosis

There have been major recent advances in understanding the molecular basis of myofibroblast activation, ECM deposition, and fibrosis. These molecules represent individual targets for anti-fibrotic therapy:

- TGF-β is the most potent stimulator of ECM production known
- The epithelial integrin $\alpha V\beta 6$ is involved in conversion of TGF-β from a latent to an activated form
- Activation of the high-affinity receptor TGFβ-R1 (also known as activin-like receptor kinase, ALK-5) results in Smad signalling
- Connective tissue growth factor (CTGF) is a downstream mediator of TGF-β
- IFN-γ downregulates RGF-β activity
- IL-13 is a strongly fibrotic Th2 cytokine that may be important in remodelling in asthma and COPD
- PDGF is a potent mitogen and differentiation factor for myofibroblasts
- CCL2 (MCP-1) and CXCL12 (ligand for CXCR4)
- PAR-2 is a transmembrane receptor preferentially activated by trypsin and tryptase, and causes the proliferation of human airway smooth muscle cells and fibroblasts.

2.5 Conclusion

Much further research is required to understand the molecular, cellular, and patho-physiological basis of COPD. It is fundamental to perform translational research on samples from patients with COPD to develop animal and human models of COPD and to study the inter-related processes of inflammation, fibrosis, and proteolysis. We need to understand better the genetics of COPD and why certain gene patterns together with a variety of environmental influences cause COPD. It is relevant to understand the molecular mechanism for the amplified inflammation characteristic of COPD, and how systemic COPD can be caused. Overall, it is necessary to understand the balance between genes and environment that is related to oxidant damage, inflammation, fibrosis, and proteolysis.

References

Barnes PJ (2008). Immunology of asthma and chronic obstructive pulmonary disease. *Nature Reviews Immunology*, **8**(3), 183–92.

Curtis JL, Freeman CM, and Hogg JC (2007). The immunopathogenesis of chronic obstructive pulmonary disease: insights from recent research 1. *Proceeding of the American Thoracic Society*, **4**(7), 512–21.

Donnelly LE and Barnes PJ (2006). Chemokine receptors as therapeutic targets in chronic obstructive pulmonary disease. *Trends in Pharmacological Sciences*, **27**(10), 546–53.

Hogg JC, Chu F, Utokaparch S et al. (2004). The nature of small-airway obstruction in chronic obstructive pulmonary disease. *The New England Journal of Medicines*, **350**(26), 2645–53.

Hogg JC (2006). State of the Art. Bronchiolitis in chronic obstructive pulmonary disease. *Proceeding of the American Thoracic Society*, **3**(6), 489–93.

Kim WD, Ling SH, Coxson HO et al. (2007). The association between small airway obstruction and emphysema phenotypes in COPD. *Chest*, **131**(5), 1372–8.

Rahman I and Adcock IM (2006). Oxidative stress and redox regulation of lung inflammation in COPD. *European Respiratory Journal*, **28**(1), 219–42.

Sabroe I and Whyte MK (2007). Toll-like receptor (TLR)-based networks regulate neutrophilic inflammation in respiratory disease. *Biochemical Society Transcations*, **35**(Pt 6), 1492–5.

Scotton CJ and Chambers RC (2007). Molecular targets in pulmonary fibrosis. lst in focus. *Chest*, **132**, 1311–21.

Vestbo J and Lange P (2002). Can GOLD Stage 0 provide information of prognostic value in chronic obstructive pulmonary disease? *American Journal of Respiratory and Critical Care Medicine*, **166**(3), 329–32.

Chapter 3

Clinical features, spirometry, and lung function

Farid Bazari, Trevor T. Hansel,
Michael I. Polkey, and Onn Min Kon

Key points

- Major indicators for considering a diagnosis of COPD are a history of (1) progressive dyspnoea on exertion, (2) a chronic productive cough, and (3) a history of exposure to risk factors.
- It is important to consider systemic features of COPD: including weight loss, muscle weakness, *cor pulmonale*, sleep abnormalities, and decreased exercise performance.
- Co-morbidities are common in COPD patients: ischaemic heart disease, carcinoma of the bronchus, depression, metabolic syndrome, endocrine abnormalities (diabetes mellitus, thyroid disorders, hypogonadism), anaemia, and osteoporosis.
- COPD is characterized by airflow obstruction with a forced expiratory volume in one second (FEV1)/forced vital capacity (FVC) ratio of <0.7.
- The FEV_1 is a predictor of mortality in COPD and useful for monitoring disease progression and response to therapy.
- Hyperinflation and air-trapping are indicated by a rise in the residual volume.
- The gas transfer is reduced in emphysema because of destruction of the alveolar-capillary membrane.
- Dynamic tests such as the 6-min walk distance can be used to assess response to therapy.

3.1 **Clinical features**

3.1.1 **History**

- Suggestive clinical features of COPD include a history of progressive shortness of breath on exertion (dyspnoea), often associated with a productive morning cough, found in a middle-aged person of more than 40 years with a long history of cigarette smoking.
- Dyspnoea is the hallmark symptom of COPD, is 'an abnormal awareness of the act of breathing', and is the main reason most COPD patients consult their doctor. The severity of dyspnoea is classified by the modified Medical Research Council (MRC) scale (see Table 3.1).
- Chronic cough is initially intermittent, but later can be present every day.
- Sputum production is not invariable and is more common after coughing bouts. Regular daily production of sputum for three or more months in two consecutive years is the epidemiological definition of 'chronic bronchitis'.
- Wheezing and chest tightness are variable non-specific symptoms.
- The patient should be questioned in detail regarding exposure to risk factors such as smoking and occupational or environmental exposures.
- In severe disease there may be weight loss, anorexia, and cachexia. Ankle swelling suggests *cor pulmonale*.
- One should carefully ask the history in the light of co-morbidities associated with smoking and COPD.

3.1.2 **Physical examination**

- Nicotine-stained fingers. Clubbing suggests a malignancy (or bronchiectasis)
- Rapid pursed lip breathing > 20 beats/min
- Use of accessory muscles of respiration: scalene and sternocleidomastpid (SCM) muscles
- Hyperinflation
  - with downward liver displacement
  - decreased crico-sternal distance
  - barrel chest
  - intercostal recession
- Central cyanosis or bluish discolouration of the mucosal membranes
- 'Pink puffers' and 'blue bloaters' have good and poor respiratory drive respectively

- Wheezing and inspiratory crackles
- *Cor pulmonale* has signs of right-sided heart failure: ankle oedema, elevated jugular venous pressure (JVP), prominent second heart sound, cardiomegaly
- Systemic COPD may have nutritional depletion with cachexia and muscle weakness and wasting.

3.1.3 **Differential diagnosis of COPD**

- Asthma
- Congestive heart failure
- Bronchiectasis
- Tuberculosis
- Obliterative bronchiolitis
- Diffuse panbronchiolitis.

3.2 **Spirometry techniques and measurement**

Simple spirometry allows for a cheap and readily available measurement of airflow (Tables 3.2 and 3.3). This is reproducible and allows assessment of airflow obstruction. Spirometry is essential for the diagnosis of COPD and allows sub-classification according to the Global Initiative for Chronic Obstructive Lung Disease (GOLD) system. There are a large variety of spirometers which range from simple portable electronic devices to the 'traditional' bellows such as the Vitalograph® series.

Grade	Level of breathlessness
\multicolumn{2}{l}{**Table 3.1 Modified MRC questionnaire for assessing the severity of breathlessness**}
0	Not troubled with breathlessness
1	Breathlessness with strenuous exertion
2	Breathless when hurrying on the level **or** Walking up a slight hill
3	Walks slower than other people of same age on the level because of breathlessness **or** Stops for breath when walking at own pace on the level
4	Stop for breath after walking about 100m **or** Breathless after a few minutes on the level
5	Too breathless to leave the house **or** Breathless when dressing or undressing

Table 3.2 Practical procedure

(i) Seat the patient.

(ii) Explain the purpose of the test.

(iii) Demonstrate the technique.

(iv) Ask the patient to take a full inspiration (i.e. filled to total lung capacity – TLC).

(v) The patient should now blow the breath out, forcibly, as hard and as fast as possible, until there is nothing left to expel—encourage the patient to keep blowing out.

(vi) Now repeat the procedure, and then repeat it again.

NB For spirometers capable of generating flow–volume loops—after a full expiration, the patient can take a rapid breath in to TLC to generate an inspiratory flow loop.

Table 3.3 Quality assurance in spirometry

Preparation

- Equipment must be regularly serviced and calibrated.
- Supervisor needs training in spirometry performance.
- Hard printed copies are needed to ensure meaningful tests.
- Maximal patient effort is required.

Performance

- It should be performed using techniques that meet required standards.
- Spirometric traces should be smooth (see examples below).
- Adequate standards are met when three reproducible tracings have been obtained with less than 150mL variability between two best measures for FEV_1 and FVC.
- The recording should be for a minimum of 6s but go on long enough for maximal FVC to be reached (may be as long as 15s in severe disease).
- FEV_1 and FVC should be taken from the maximal of three tracings.
- FEV_1/FVC ratio should be taken from the technically best curve and maximal recordings.

The manoeuvre is performed with the patient sitting and repeated on three occasions to obtain reproducible and reliable readings. Spirometry is dependent on patient effort and therefore requires strict instruction and observation by a trained individual. As with all lung function, accurate calibration and maintenance of equipment is important. Data are usually expressed at body temperature (BTPS) rather than ambient temperature (ATPS; usually assumed to be 23°C).

3.2.1 Measurements

The volume of air exhaled over 1s from a full inspiration is defined as the forced expiratory volume in 1s (FEV_1). The total volume of air expired at the end of expiration (may be as long as 15s in COPD) is defined as the forced vital capacity (FVC).

The ratio of the FEV_1/FVC is calculated. A ratio of <70% is defined as airflow obstruction and is essential for a diagnosis of COPD. The

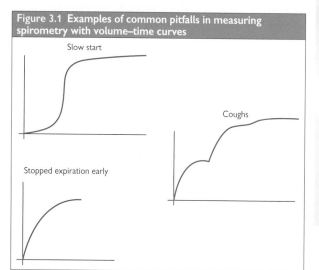

Figure 3.1 Examples of common pitfalls in measuring spirometry with volume–time curves

Slow start

Coughs

Stopped expiration early

absolute values of FEV_1 and FVC are compared with reference values according to the patient's age, sex, height, and ethnic origin.

When reviewing spirometric data, it is useful to assess both the flow versus volume curve, as well as volume versus time curve as they give more accurate visual indices of the beginning and end of expiration respectively (Figures 3.1 and 3.3).

3.3 Spirometric definition of COPD

COPD is characterized by poorly reversible airflow limitation. One must demonstrate evidence of airflow obstruction in order to make a diagnosis of COPD. This means that the FEV_1 is proportionally reduced compared to the FVC. (equating to an FEV_1/FVC ratio of less than 0.7). There is usually an absolute reduction in FEV_1 (as compared with a reference range based on height, age, sex, and ethnicity) of less than 80% predicted, but the FVC may be preserved. The degree of airflow limitation may then be classified according to % predicted FEV_1, which has a prognostic effect on all-cause mortality in COPD (Figure 3.2).

It should be pointed out that as the process of aging does affect lung volumes there is a possibility of the over-diagnosis of COPD in the elderly using the fixed FEV_1/FVC ratio (Figure 3.2). There is therefore a pressing need to develop verifiable 'normal' post-bronchodilator values in the elderly.

Figure 3.2 Spirometry in COPD

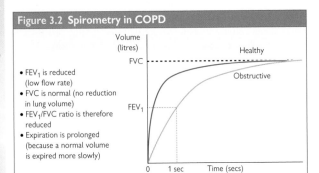

- FEV$_1$ is reduced (low flow rate)
- FVC is normal (no reduction in lung volume)
- FEV$_1$/FVC ratio is therefore reduced
- Expiration is prolonged (because a normal volume is expired more slowly)

Figure 3.3 Flow–volume loop for COPD

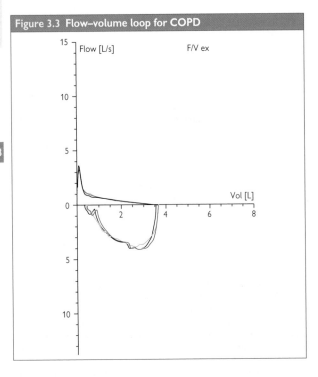

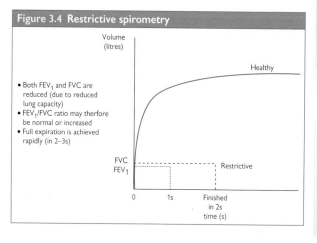

Figure 3.4 Restrictive spirometry

Volume
(litres)

Healthy

- Both FEV$_1$ and FVC are
  reduced (due to reduced
  lung capacity)
- FEV$_1$/FVC ratio may therfore
  be normal or increased
- Full expiration is achieved
  rapidly (in 2–3s)

FVC
FEV$_1$ Restrictive

0   1s   Finished
                          in 2s
                          time (s)

3.4 Spirometry: indications for use

Spirometry should be performed when any patient is suspected to
have COPD. For example, smokers or ex-smokers aged >35 years
with cough, sputum, breathlessness, frequent winter bronchitis, or
wheeze.

Spirometry can be useful in narrowing down the list of differential
diagnoses causing the patient's symptoms. A restrictive spirometry
(FEV$_1$/FVC > 0.7 and proportionately reduced FVC) may be seen in
conditions affecting lung parenchyma such as idiopathic pulmonary
fibrosis or those affecting the muscles such as neuromuscular disease
(see Figure 3.4).

3.5 Bronchodilator reversibility (BDR) testing

Bronchodilator testing is not performed routinely; however, when it
is performed it should be done under strict conditions. In cases
where asthma (rather than COPD) is suspected as the cause of symptoms, bronchodilator reversibility testing is recommended (Table 3.4).
Demonstration of variable airflow obstruction, as well as bronchodilator
reversibility (BDR), points strongly to a diagnosis of asthma (Figure 3.5).
By definition, COPD demonstrates poorly reversible airflow obstruction.
A lack of any bronchodilator response does not predict the efficacy of
any bronchodilator in COPD and therefore BDR should not be used
to define treatment.

Table 3.4 **BDR testing: instructions**

- Patient should withhold all bronchodilators prior to the test if possible. No short-acting bronchodilator for 6h, no long-acting bronchodilator for 12h, no long-acting oral theophylline for 24h.
- Perform baseline spirometry (best of three readings).
- Administer short-acting inhaled bronchodilator.
- Repeat spirometry 15min later (best of three readings).
- Calculate the percentage and absolute change in FEV_1 and FVC. An absolute FEV_1 rise of 200mL and 15% relative rise are defined as reversible; however, it should be noted that reversibility is a spectrum of response rather than an 'all or nothing phenomenon'.

Figure 3.5 **BDR testing in asthma and COPD**

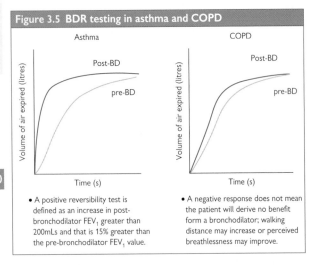

- A positive reversibility test is defined as an increase in post-bronchodilator FEV_1 greater than 200mLs and that is 15% greater than the pre-bronchodilator FEV_1 value.

- A negative response does not mean the patient will derive no benefit form a bronchodilator; walking distance may increase or perceived breathlessness may improve.

3.6 **Spirometric classification of COPD**

There are a number of severity classifications using FEV_1. For the purposes of this chapter we will look at the GOLD guidelines. Note that other classifications are also provided by bodies such as the American Thoracic Society (ATS). Importantly the criteria in use in the United Kingdom provided by NICE do not recognize the mildest of the GOLD criteria (see Table 3.5).

COPD severity is graded according to the demonstrated degree of airflow obstruction, as measured by post-bronchodilator FEV_1. This has prognostic implications for both morbidity and mortality.

Table 3.5 GOLD spirometric classification of COPD severity based on post-bronchodilator FEV_1

	GOLD spirometric classification of COPD severity based on post-bronchodilator FEV_1	NICE spirometric guidelines for COPD (note lack of mild group with $FEV_1 > 80\%$)
Stage I	Mild $FEV_1/FVC < 0.70$ $FEV_1 > 80\%$ predicted	Mild, FEV_1 50–80%
Stage II	Moderate $FEV_1/FVC < 0.70$ FEV_1 50–80% predicted	Moderate, FEV_1 30–49%
Stage III	Severe $FEV_1/FVC < 0.70$ FEV_1 30–50% predicted	Severe, $FEV_1 < 30\%$
Stage IV	Very Severe $FEV_1/FVC < 0.70$ $FEV_1 < 30\%$ predicted or $FEV_1 < 50\%$ predicted plus chronic respiratory failure (i.e. $pO_2 < 7.3$ mmHg or $pCO_2 > 6$ mmHg)	

3.7 Spirometry as a tool for monitoring disease progress and treatment response

Smoking is associated with a more rapid rate of decline of FEV_1. In view of the ease of measurement and prognostic significance, the rate of decline of FEV_1 is used as a marker of treatment success in a number of trials. Drug studies that have demonstrated a slowing in the rate of decline of or increase in FEV_1 are then used as evidence of efficacy of these therapies.

Spirometry is also used in the outpatient clinic as an additional tool to assess individual patient's response to novel therapies.

Along with body-mass index, 6-min walk distance, and breathlessness scores as defined by MRC grade, FEV_1 provides additional prognostic information in assessing patients with known COPD.

The limitations of FEV_1 as a single measure must be noted as it only assesses the degree of airflow obstruction in COPD and not the effect of this disease on other systems. In addition, it does not provide any measure of gas transfer, hyperinflation (which may affect lung mechanics), or the performance of the lungs during exercise. For this we need more detailed testing of lung function at rest or during exercise.

3.8 **Other measures of lung function in COPD**

3.8.1 **Body plethysmography**

Body plethysmography is the gold standard measure for static lung volumes. This involves breathing against a closed shutter and works on the assumption that in a closed circuit pressure at the mouth equates to that of the airways.

Body plethysmography is of value in COPD in giving extra information compared to simple spirometry. Static lung volumes (Figure 3.6) which can be calculated using this technique include the residual volume (RV) and TLC.

Measurement of RV is important in COPD, as it signifies the degree of hyperinflation. The RV is the volume of air left in the lungs at the end of a complete expiratory manoeuvre. In COPD, the RV is increased, as the collapse of small airways during expiration prevents the emptying of alveoli. The subsequent hyperinflation interferes with lung mechanics, thus increasing the work of breathing.

Figure 3.6 **Static lung volumes**

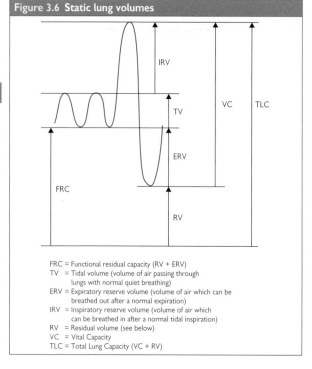

FRC = Functional residual capacity (RV + ERV)
TV = Tidal volume (volume of air passing through lungs with normal quiet breathing)
ERV = Expiratory reserve volume (volume of air which can be breathed out after a normal expiration)
IRV = Inspiratory reserve volume (volume of air which can be breathed in after a normal tidal inspiration)
RV = Residual volume (see below)
VC = Vital Capacity
TLC = Total Lung Capacity (VC + RV)

3.8.2 Gas-transfer measurement

The diffusion capacity of the lungs estimates the transfer of oxygen from the alveoli to the red blood cell. It is estimated using a single breath hold of 10s using carbon monoxide (CO) and is termed the transfer factor of the lung for CO (TLCO) by the European community and diffusing capacity of the lung for CO (DLCO) by the North American community.

It is reduced in conditions that disrupt the alveolar-capillary surface area. In emphysema, where there is destruction of the alveolar-capillary surface area in addition to an obstructive defect, there is reduced gas transfer contributing to dyspnoea.

It should be noted that there is significant inter-laboratory variation in absolute gas-transfer measurements and hence values are also expressed as the percentage predicted of normal. Secondary polycythaemia is common in COPD and if uncorrected may cause TLCO and KCO (coefficient of gas transfer) measurements to appear falsely normal/high. Ideally a measure of the haemoglobin by a haemocytometer within the laboratory is performed to correct the value

3.8.3 Six-minute walk distance

This is a dynamic test of exercise capacity under controlled conditions. The subject walks 6min in a 100-foot hallway marked out with 'turn-around' cones. They choose their own pace and can stop for a rest during the test. This is a good reflection of activities of daily living as it is performed at sub-maximal pace.

The 6-min walk distance is a useful disease marker in COPD both at baseline and as a measure of response to therapy, such as lung volume reduction surgery. It also correlates well with quality of life scores and is an independent predictor of mortality. It is useful in measuring dynamic hyperinflation which occurs during exercise and thus correlates with reduced exercise capacity.

It is essential to note that dynamic hyperinflation contributes significantly to dyspnoea during exercise in patients who may otherwise be classified as those with mild disease (GOLD Stage 1). Dynamic hyperinflation is a consequence of the inability to increase expiratory flow at normal end-expiratory volumes, which during exercise (increased respiratory rate) leads to worsening hyperinflation. This in turn increases the work of breathing and leads to reduced exercise capacity and dyspnoea. Dynamic hyperinflation can be measured by inspiratory capacity during exercise. It correlates with dyspnoea during exercise and exercise limitation.

3.8.4 Cardio-pulmonary exercise testing (CPET)

A more formal measure of exercise capacity is obtained using CPET. The advantage of this method is that it allows one to measure the cardio-respiratory performance during exercise. This will allow assessment of all the systems involved in exercise, including respiratory function, cardiovascular function, right heart and pulmonary circulation, as well as muscle function.

CPET has many indications, including investigation of the breathless patient where no identifiable cause has been found. It is of value in pre-operative assessment of patients with significant cardio-respiratory disease. It is also used as a pre-operative assessment tool for patients with significant COPD who need to undergo surgery for resection of a lung neoplasm, where an oxygen uptake of <15mL/min/kg is associated with an increased risk.

The availability and use of CPET is limited, although there is a clear role for its use in assessing dynamic cardio-respiratory function. In the routine setting, the 6-min walk distance has good correlation with maximal oxygen delivery (vO_2 max) and is obviously much more available.

Key reference

National Institute for Health (NIH), National Heart Lung and Blood Institute of the USA (NHLBI), and the World Health Organization (WHO), Global Initiative for Chronic Obstructive Lung Disease (GOLD): Global strategy for the diagnosis, management, and prevention of COPD. http://www.goldcopd.org, Updated in 2007.

References

(2001). Dynamic hyperinflation and exercise intolerance in chronic obstructive pulmonary disease. *American Journal of Respiratory and Critical Care Medicine.* **164**(5), 770–7.

(2001). Inspiratory capacity, dynamic hyperinflation, breathlessness, and exercise performance during the 6-minute-walk test in chronic obstructive pulmonary disease. *American Journal of Respiratory and Critical Care Medicine.* **163** (6), 1395–9.

(2001). Lower respiratory illnesses promote FEV_1 decline in current smokers but not ex-smokers with mild chronic obstructive pulmonary disease; Results from the Lung Health Study. *American Journal of Respiratory and Critical Care Medicine.* **164** (3), 358–64.

(2000). Pulmonary function is a predictor of long term mortality in the general population, 29 year follow-up of Buffalo Health Study. *Chest.* **118**, 656–64.

(2005). Standardization of Spirometry, *The European Respiratory Journal.* **26**, 319–38.

(2004). The body-mass index, airflow obstruction, dyspnea, and exercise capacity index in chronic obstructive pulmonary disease. *NEJM.* **350**, 1005–12.

Chapter 4

Imaging in COPD

Onn Min Kon and Aimee L. Brame

Key points
• Plain chest X-rays are normal in mild COPD.
• Increased bronchovascular markings on chest X-rays are seen in chronic bronchitis.
• Hyperinflation, bullae, and oligaemia are seen in chest X-rays in emphysema.
• High-resolution computed tomography (HRCT) scans are useful for detecting, defining the extent, and distribution of emphysema.
• High-resolution CT scans allow for discrimination of COPD from other pulmonary diseases.

4.1 Introduction

Although COPD is a functional diagnosis, imaging can play an important role in the assessment of patients with COPD. However, two of the major components of the disease, chronic bronchitis and emphysema, do not 'lend themselves equally to imaging' and will be addressed separately. We will briefly discuss the radiological abnormalities found in respiratory bronchiolitis-associated interstitial lung disease (RBILD). Other disorders which are characterized by airflow obstruction, such as asthma and bronchiectasis, are beyond the remit of this chapter.

4.2 Imaging in chronic bronchitis

Chronic bronchitis is defined in clinical terms, as 'a chronic or recurrent increase in the volume of mucoid bronchial secretions sufficient to cause expectoration and occurring on most days for three months in two or more successive years'. The major pathological change in chronic bronchitis is mucous gland hypertrophy and hyperplasia in the large airways. Patients with chronic bronchitis may have normal pulmonary function tests. The radiographic features are non-specific, and the chest radiograph is often normal—any abnormalities which may be seen are subtle and non-specific.

4.2.1 Described features on plain radiograph

These include:

- Hyperinflation (with co-existent emphysema)
- Increased lung markings, ill-defined linear densities
- Minor areas of fibrosis
- Thickened bronchial walls, either in cross section 'ring shadows', or in longitudinal section as 'tram lines'
- If pulmonary hypertension has developed—enlarged central pulmonary arteries
- Superadded pathology—pneumonia, pneumothoraces, pulmonary oedema, mass lesions.

4.2.2 CT findings in chronic bronchitis

These are non-specific.
Abnormalities described in the literature include:

- Bronchial wall thickening
- Interlobular septal thickening
- Mucous plugging of bronchioles
- Peripheral tree-in-bud
- Air-trapping
- Central arterial dilatation reflecting pulmonary hypertension
- Mild mediastinal lymphadenopathy consistent with chronic low-grade infection.

4.3 Imaging in emphysema

Emphysema is defined as a condition of the lung characterized by 'abnormal permanent enlargement of the air spaces distal to the terminal bronchiole, accompanied by destruction of their walls without obvious fibrosis'. In contrast to bronchitis, it is a pathological rather than a clinical diagnosis.

There are four major patterns of emphysema, defined anatomically as:

1. Centrilobular—affecting the respiratory bronchioles in the central portion of the lobule, usually upper zone, associated with smoking
2. Panlobular—uniform enlargement and destruction of the entire lobule, seen in alpha 1 anti-trypsin deficiency with post-bronchiolar obstruction

3. Paraseptal—the peripheral part of the lobule is selectively involved, often subpleural, also around interlobular septa and fissures. Air spaces can become confluent and develop into bullae
4. Irregular—around scars, often associated with fibrosis.

4.3.1 Plain chest radiography in emphysema

This may be normal in mild disease. In severe disease the following abnormalities can be seen.

- Hyperinflation:
  - Low diaphragm—characterized by the dome of the diaphragm lying less than 1.5cm above straight line drawn from costophrenic junction and vertebrophrenic junction
  - Flat diaphragm—defined as mid point of right hemidiaphragm below or at the level of the anterior end of the seventh rib
  - Widened retrosternal airspace (space between ascending aorta and sternum, 3cm below the manubrium) more than 2.5cm on lateral film
  - Retrosternal airspace extending down to within 3cm of the diaphragm on a lateral film
  - Costophrenic angle of more than 90 degrees on a lateral radiograph
  - Narrow cardiac silhouette, with lung markings visible through the heart.
- Vascular
  - Number and size of pulmonary vessels and branches are reduced in the middle and outer regions of the lung
  - Rapid tapering and attenuation of vessels
  - Distorted, tortuous, or abnormally straight vessels, widened branching angles, and loss of side branches
  - Emphysema has a patchy distribution; more prominent vessels may be apparent in normal lung because of compensatory engorgement.
  - Demarcated, avascular areas, representing bullae.
- Bullae—sharply demarcated thin walled area of emphysema, more than 1cm diameter. Avascular, with surrounding atelectasis .

4.3.2 Computed tomography (CT) findings in emphysema

Plain radiography is unreliable in mild to moderate disease, and even in severe disease signs are often subject to considerable differences in interpretation (Figure 4.1). In contrast, CT (in particular high-resolution CT [HRCT]) has proved to be very sensitive and specific in detecting, localizing, characterizing, assessing, and grading emphysema.

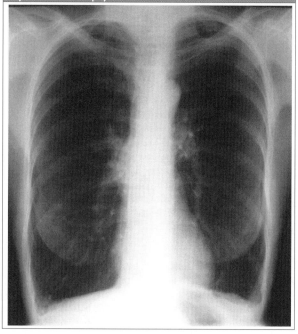

Figure 4.1 Hyperinflated lungs on plain chest radiograph in patient with emphysema

CT allows us to quantify emphysema using assessments of tissue density, visualize the lung, localize the abnormalities, and assess volume, blood flow, and other pulmonary pathology.

CT quantification of the extent and severity of emphysema can be used to map and therefore monitor the progression of the disease and evaluate any treatment.

CT scans can be assessed by subjective visual methods, density measurements, or more recently, by image processing and texture analysis. There is no Global Initiative for Chronic Obstructive Lung Disease (GOLD) standard for measuring the extent of emphysema, although studies have shown good correlation between macroscopic pathology scores (the current standard) and HRCT visual assessment.

Emphysema is characterized by focal abnormal collections of air and therefore can be assessed by measuring lung density. CT lung density is related to the amount of air, tissue, interstitial fluid, and blood within a given area, known as a voxel. Areas with higher density appear whiter on the CT scan; areas containing air appear blacker. The assessment of lung density by CT can be affected by state of inflation of the lung, gravity, interstitial fluid, position, and so forth.

HRCT is defined as thin section CT optimized by using an edge enhancing algorithm. HRCT closely reflects gross pathological findings and has the best sensitivity and specificity of any imaging method for the assessment of focal and diffuse lung diseases. Subjective CT quantification of emphysema is based on the visual assessment of area of vascular disruption and decreased attenuation in comparison with normal parenchyma. Objective CT assessment of emphysema requires computer scoring of attenuation values of the CT images. At a given threshold for soft-tissue lung interface, lung tissue is separated from the thoracic wall and the mediastinum by semi-automatic contour tracing. The lung itself is then analysed. Frequency data for each pixel attenuation value (Hounsfield unit, HU) is generated. This creates a graph known as a CT lung density histogram. This can then be used to assess severity of disease based on either percentiles of pixels below certain densities or percentage of lung volume below a given HU. In this way HRCT is able to distinguish emphysema from normal lungs even in the mildest degrees. This can then be used to monitor progression of disease.

Recent years have seen the advancement of CT from one detector to multidetector CT (multislice) scanning, improving resolution, and decreasing artefact, whilst decreasing scanning time. Spiral CT provides continuous scanning whilst the patient is being moved through the CT scanner; it has the major advantage that the entire thorax is imaged in a single breath hold. It has replaced the slice-by-slice acquisition of conventional CT. From spiral CT data, 3D reconstructions in any plane, lung volume measurements, and quantification of lung disorders can be obtained. With the use of graphics software, spiral CT data can be used to depict the luminal surfaces of the airways in a way that resemble bronchoscopy or bronchography ('virtual bronchoscopy'). In combination with IV contrast, spiral CT becomes a CT pulmonary angiograph, allowing visualization of pulmonary vessels.

Centrilobular emphysema is characterized on HRCT by the presence of multiple small round areas of abnormally low attenuation, several millimetres to a centimetre in diameter, usually with an upper lobe predominance, but can be distributed throughout the lung (Figure 4.2). The low-density areas are typically focal, remote from the pleura, and related to centrilobular arteries. The lucencies tend to be multiple, small, and 'spotty', giving a rather 'moth eaten' appearance. Classically, the areas of attenuation in centrilobular emphysema lack walls. The lung surrounding these areas looks normal; with disease progression, the lesions become more confluent.

In *panlobular emphysema* destruction is more uniform, and gives rise to generalized low-density areas and is characterized by the presence of fewer, and smaller than normal vessels—it may be diffuse, but is almost always more severe in the lower lobes (Figure 4.3). In severe

Figure 4.2 Centrilobular emphysema on CT

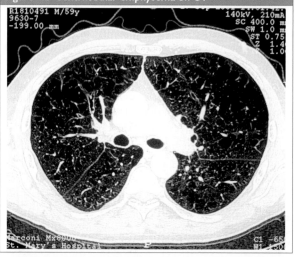

Figure 4.3 Panlobular basal emphysema in a patient with α-1 anti-trypsin deficiency

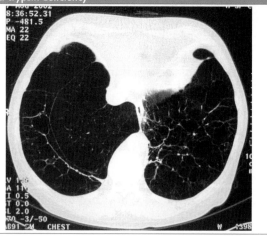

disease, extensive parenchymal destruction is easily identified, but in mild to moderate disease increased parenchymal lucency and slightly smaller vessel diameter may be missed.

Paraseptal emphysema is easily detected on HRCT (Figure 4.4). Multiple areas of subpleural or peri-fissural emphysema are seen, often with thin walls corresponding to interlobular septa. Emphysematous change may also be seen in relation to the bronchovascular bundles, in the azygoesophageal recess or adjacent to the heart border. Subpleural bullae may also be seen. The surrounding lung is normal.

Dependent ground-glass opacification is seen in some patients with emphysema. It is due to the patchy nature of the disease allowing some lobules to partially collapse, increasing their attenuation. Unlike pathological ground-glass shadowing, dependent atelectasis will resolve with change in position, if there is doubt, the scan should be repeated in the prone position.

Other features of severe emphysema include:

- Apposition of the right and left lung in the retrosternal region as a result of hyperinflation

Figure 4.4 Paraseptal emphysema on CT

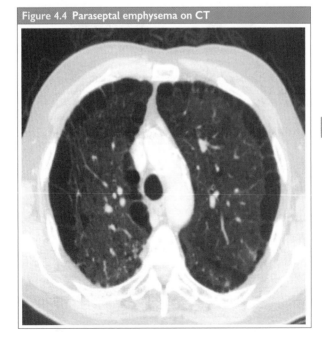

- An increased distance between the sternum and the aorta of more than 4cm corresponds to the increased retrosternal space seen on Chest X-ray and is a marker of hyperinflation

Emphysema is characterized by permanent enlargement of airspaces. CT assessment in full inspiration is more accurate for quantifying emphysema

In full expiration, gas-trapping, and airway obstruction are clearer. The differential diagnosis for emphysema include:

- Pulmonary fibrosis with honeycombing—however, the cysts are smaller and are associated with fibrosis
- Pneumatoceles—identical to bullae, but transient and related to infection
- Cystic lung disease—multiple cysts with distinct walls
- Obliterative bronchiolitis—small airways disease with patchy distribution and associated with bronchiectasis.

In mild to moderate disease, HRCT can easily differentiate the various types of emphysema—as the severity increases, this differentiation is lost.

It also has a role in treatment of disease with lung volume reduction providing knowledge of the location of lesions and is able to objectively aid surgical decision making.

4.3.3 **Tracheal abnormalities**

The cross-sectional area of the trachea can be described by the tracheal index – a ration of the coronal and sagittal diameters of the trachea. A sabre-sheath trachea is defined as a tracheal index of less than 0.6 measured 1cm above the upper margin of the aortic arch. A possible cause for the sabre-sheath trachea is air-trapping in the upper lobes related to centrilobular emphysema.

4.4 **Imaging in RBILD**

Respiratory bronchiolitis is a very common incidental finding in cigarette smokers, consisting of an accumulation of pigmented macrophages within respiratory bronchioles and adjacent alveoli. In a small portion of smokers, symptomatic interstitial lung disease may occur in association with this lesion—respiratory bronchiolitis-associated interstitial lung disease (RBILD). RBILD can be viewed as an exaggerated respiratory bronchiolitic response resulting in cough, shortness of breath, and pulmonary function impairment. This is a clinicopathological entity that may be confused with other interstitial lung diseases, in particular, idiopathic pulmonary fibrosis (IPF). In mild to moderate disease, a period of observation after smoking cessation is usually warranted to allow spontaneous regression of disease, as almost always occurs in patients with respiratory bronchiolitis.

Abnormalities in chest radiographs in RBILD include patchy ground-glass shadowing and bronchial wall thickening.

HRCT findings in RBILD:

- Areas of ground-glass attenuation—it has been postulated that the areas of ground-glass attenuation reflect 'smoker's alveolitis'
- Centrilobular ill-defined micronodules (2–3mm)—represent respiratory bronchiolitis
- Associated emphysematous changes may be present.

4.5 **Future modalities in COPD imaging**

The main developments in magnetic resonance (MR) imaging have been the introduction of MR angiography and functional MR ventilation imaging. MRI using hyperpolarized helium 3 gas has emerged as a new method for assessing pulmonary physiology, structure, and function. Using inhaled agents which can be visualized as contrast media, ventilation defects can be detected. MRA consists of 3D single breath hold images using gadolinium-based contrast agents, and may potentially have a role in detection of pulmonary emboli.

Functional MR ventilation imaging may allow assessment of regional ventilation as well as evaluation of regional oxygen partial pressures and V/Q ratios. MR allows assessment of global lung function, such as measurement of inspiratory and expiratory lung volumes as well as regional lung function, such as ventilation per unit volume at the lobar, segmental, or subsegmental level. It allows simultaneous measurement of lung perfusion. In comparison with CT scanning, the resolution is lower; however, MR has the advantage that it is radiation free, and can provide information about a broad range of functional parameters such as regional oxygen tension and ventilation/perfusion ratios. MR may provide higher sensitivity that CT, scintigraphy, or lung function tests in the diagnosis of ventilation defects. Further research is required.

References

Calverly PMA, MacNee W, Pride NB, and Rennard SI (eds) (2003). *Chronic obstructive pulmonary disease*, 2nd edition. Hodder Arnold, London.

De Jong PA, Muller NL, Pare PD, and Coxson HO (2005). Computed tomographic imaging of the airways: relationship to structure and function. *The European Respiratory Journal*, **26**, 140–152.

Hansell DM, Armstrong P, Lynch DA, McAdams HP (2005). *Disease of the airways*, 4th edition. Mosby, London.

Hansell DM (2001). Small airways diseases: detection and insights with computed tomography. *The European Respiratory Journal*, **17**, 1294–1313.

Madani A, Keyser C, and Gevenois PA (2001). Quantitative computed tomography assessment of lung structure and function in pulmonary emphysema. *The European Respiratory Journal* **18**, 720–30.

McCloud TC (1998). *Thoracic Radiology: the Requisites*. Mosby, St. Louis.

Muller NL (2001), Advances in imaging. *The European Respiratory Journal*, **18**, 867–71.

Reed JC (2003). Chest radiology: plain film patterns and differential diagnoses, 5th edition. Mosby, Philadelphia, Pa,.

Stavngaard T, Sogaard LV, Mortensen J, *et al.* (2005). Hyperpolarised ^{3}HeMRI and ^{81m}Kr SPECT in chronic obstructive pulmonary disease. *European Journal of Nuclear Medicine*, **32**(4), 448–57.

Chapter 5

Smoking cessation

Susannah A.A. Bloch and Onn Min Kon

- Smoking cessation is currently the only intervention that causes a slowing in the natural history of an accelerated loss of forced expiratory volume in 1s (FEV_1) in COPD.
- The addictive properties of nicotine in tobacco are mediated primarily through the release of dopamine in the nucleus accumbens via nicotinic receptors.
- Smoking advice should be carried out regularly by all health professionals and has been shown to be effective.
- Both behavioural therapy and pharmacological therapies have been shown to be effective in achieving smoking cessation.
- Nicotine replacement, bupropion, and varenicline are first-line agents that increase the likelihood of successful smoking cessation.

5.1 Background

Although there are other factors associated with the risk of developing COPD, smoking is by far the commonest cause of this disease—usually occurring after a smoking history of more than 20 pack-years. However, the risks of smoking do not relate just to COPD, and UK government data collected between 1988 and 2002 showed that on average 90,000 deaths per year can be attributed to smoking, hence making it one of the major causes of preventable deaths. With respect to COPD the natural loss in forced expiratory volume in 1s (FEV_1) which usually occurs with age occurs at an accelerated rate in those smokers who develop COPD. Smoking cessation is so far the only intervention that can slow this progressive loss of lung function.

The positive effects of smoking cessation have been described in several landmark studies. The Fletcher and Peto study demonstrated in a cohort of 792 working men that over the course of 8yrs smoking cessation resulted in a decline in the rate of loss of FEV_1 per year, which although not returning their lung function to baseline, reverted the decline to that of the non-smoking rate. The longest study conducted was 'The Smoking Doctors' study which followed patients over a course of 50 years and was able to demonstrate that smoking cessation at all ages is still beneficial. If persuaded to stop by 50 the risks associated with smoking were almost halved and if smokers quit by age 30 the risk was avoided. Even at 60 stopping smoking resulted in a mean increase in survival of 3 years compared to that of continuing smokers. A randomized controlled study of 5887 early COPD patients carried out between 1986 and 1994 in North America to assess the efficacy of smoking cessation also showed that smoking cessation slowed the rate of decline in FEV_1.

A survey of smokers showed that 73% wish to stop smoking, with most stating at least one potential health advantage for stopping smoking. However, only 2–3% of smokers quit permanently each year. Although at least half of such smokers have tried to quit within the last year, success rates are low. There are psychosocial factors that continue to promote smoking, and there is evidence of a trend towards people of a younger age starting to smoke as well as an increase in the proportion of young females taking up smoking. However, nicotine is likely to be the major factor in causing individuals to start and maintain tobacco addiction.

5.2 **Neurobiology of nicotine**

Nicotine acts through multiple neurotransmitters including dopamine, noradrenaline, 5-hydroxytryptamine, glutamate, gamma-aminobutyric acid (GABA), and even endogenous opioid peptides. The receptors for nicotine in the brain are the nicotinic acetylcholine receptors (nACh). High- and low-affinity nACh receptors are found in the mesocorticolimbic dopaminergic neurons. There are low nACh receptors found in the hippocampus and cortex. Dopamine release by nicotine is linked to the reward centre in the nucleus accumbens. When a smoker stops smoking nicotine withdrawal causes nicotine 'hunger'. This goes from the simple urge to smoke to more pronounced physical and psychological symptoms, with depression and mood swings being common features. Nicotine withdrawal is the main reason that many attempts to quit are unsuccessful, because the above unpleasant symptoms are relieved by smoking again. Nicotine withdrawal starts within about 20min of the last cigarette, peaking at about 72h and then subsiding over the next two weeks to a month The complex interaction between 'positive' and 'negative' addictive effects of nicotine exposure and then the positive social reinforcements when one smokes adds to the real dilemma of smoking cessation not being able to be solved by just a pure pharmacological approach.

5.3 Psychological/cognitive approaches

Psychological and cognitive approaches to smoking cessation take many different forms, and their success probably depends on the individuals involved. Self-help material is readily available in many different forms—when compared to no intervention it is difficult to prove that it is beneficial. However, more formal psychological interventions have strong evidence bases behind their use.

5.3.1 Brief advice

There is good evidence that brief advice offered by physicians or nurses can provide a small but significant effect of about 2.5% of patients quitting. Brief advice is defined as a 5–10min discussion with a non-specially trained health professional, and it is suggested that individuals will be more receptive to this when it is linked to their current health problem, but that any further intervention should be carried out by a specially trained professional. Also it is important to recognize that repeat attempts at brief advice may be detrimental. It has also been recently demonstrated that telling smokers their lung age significantly improves the likelihood of them quitting smoking.

5.3.2 Counselling

Individual counselling has been demonstrated to be effective, with evidence that the length of such sessions has a dose response .Group counselling allows several individuals to be helped by an individual therapist and may be more cost-effective. This approach has the advantage of not only teaching behavioural techniques but also supplying mutual support. Proactive telephone counselling has advantages over standard self-help programmes but does not offer any advantage over and above pharmacotherapy with or without face to face counselling.

Most trials of smoking cessation medications include psychological support measures, and when comparing medication versus support or combined, the combination has the greatest effect. For example, a large trial in the United States achieved 25% quit rates at 1yr when combining nicotine replacement therapy with intensive protracted behavioural support.

5.4 Pharmacological approaches

5.4.1 Nicotine replacement approaches

Nicotine replacement therapy (NRT) is based on the theory that maintaining nicotine levels in the body allows withdrawal symptoms to be minimized and therefore smoking behaviour to be gradually stopped. NRT is currently available in many forms such as gum, sprays, patches, and inhalators. A Cochrane review evaluated

132 trials directly comparing nicotine replacement with placebo and
showed an overall odds ratio for abstinence of 1.58. However, no one
preparation was more successful than others. There was evidence
that 4mg gum had better efficacy than a 2mg preparation in heavily
dependent smokers. It is recommended that heavier smokers use the
stronger preparations. In addition, even the most rapidly absorbed
NRT preparation cannot achieve the peak plasma concentrations of
nicotine that smoking achieves. Nicotine replacement methods can
be used alone or in combination. Using a patch to deal with back-
ground withdrawal and a more short-acting preparation (such as a
nasal spray) for breakthrough urges have been shown to be more
effective. NRT is normally weaned off after a period of about 12 weeks.
Light smokers may experience very strong urges rather than withdrawal and therefore short-acting preparations should be used.
There is evidence from subgroup analysis that nicotine replacement
is as successful in light as heavy smokers. However, a randomized
controlled trial of just light smokers on NRT in comparison to placebo
only showed a non-significant improvement. Nicotine replacement
is also licensed to help people cut down their daily number of
cigarettes—this is advised when people are not yet ready to quit,
but are keen to reduce their tobacco intake with an overall goal of
eventually giving up.

There is interest in the apparent relative safety of non-smoked
tobacco (such as snus used in Sweden), and this may be a possible
alternative NRT preparation in the future although currently this is
not legally available in many parts of Europe.

5.4.2 Antidepressants

It is thought that nicotine may have antidepressant properties that
help to maintain smoking. The antidepressants bupropion and
nortriptyline have evidence from large meta-analysis that they are
effective. The Cochrane database looked at 40 trials for bupropion
and 8 for nortriptyline and found that both can approximately double
cessation rate (odds ratio of 1.94 for bupropion, 2.32 for nortriptyline). However, in the United Kingdom only bupropion is licensed
for smoking cessation. At the moment there is not enough evidence
to suggest that nicotine replacement and antidepressants should
be used together. These odds ratios are similar to those found for
nicotine replacement and there is no evidence to support one
modality over the other currently. Unfortunately both bupropion
and nortryptiline are associated with significant side effects, for
example nausea and anxiety. Generally people should be advised that
these abate within the first few weeks, but approximately 2% of
people do stop taking them because of these side effects. Serious
side effects are rare but include a 1 in 1000 risk of seizures—this is
similar with all antidepressants.

5.4.3 Varenicline

Varenicline is licensed for use in smokers who have expressed a desire to quit and is a partial agonist to the α_4 β_2 nicotine receptor. Hence it reduces symptoms of withdrawal (by partial release of dopamine) and also decreases the rewarding effects of smoking by blocking the receptor. A meta-analysis of such trials have shown increased effectiveness when compared with placebo (odds ratio 3.2), buproprion and nicotine replacement therapy. Many of these studies followed up smokers for up to 52 weeks and still found statistically significant results at these time points. Notably most of these studies included regular and continued psychological support, which may have helped increase the overall success rate seen. The standard course of varenicline is 9–12 weeks, but some trials continued treatment for 24 weeks, starting 1–2 weeks prior to an agreed quit date. With a prolonged course the chance or relapse at 6 months may also be reduced by as much as 30%. Side effects are mainly abdominal, nausea, and diarrhoea. Overall, varenicline is thought to be safe and effective and has recently been added to the list of therapies recommended by NICE for smoking cessation.

5.4.4 Developing therapies

Rimonabant (a CB1 receptor antagonist) was initially developed as a drug to help weight loss; when its ability to help smoking cessation was suggested it appeared that these combined effects would have great potential to stop smoking and prevent post-cessation weight gain. However, since then there have been questions raised about its safety (with respect to depression and suicidal ideation), and this has therefore not received a license for smoking cessation. Nicotine vaccines are also being developed, and some are already being evaluated in clinical trials. Currently there are three nicotine vaccinations being evaluated, and this is achieved by either binding the molecule with a carrier protein, virus-like particle, or cholera toxin. The vaccine should theoretically result in the binding of nicotine with antibodies, hence rendering the bound molecule too large to cross the blood brain barrier and thus preventing binding to central nicotine receptors. This in theory should reduce nicotine's pleasurable and addictive effects.

5.5 Alternative therapies

Hypnosis, the Alan Carr method, aversion therapy (rapid smoking), and acupuncture are amongst the alternative therapies currently available to the public and proposed as aids to help people stop smoking. However, some of these approaches may be expensive, and, in addition, these generally advise against the use of medications, which is counter to most national guidance. These approaches have been shown on meta-analyses to be non-efficacious, or in some cases there are no clinical data to be able to judge their efficacy.

5.6 Conclusion

Health professionals dealing with COPD patients need to use every opportunity to promote smoking cessation as this is the single most important intervention in COPD. There are now a variety of proven approaches and this is best as a combination of cognitive and pharmacological therapies. However, it is recognized that with even the most encouraging studies, showing successful quit rates of only about 25%, there is still a significant amount of novel drug development that is required to improve the chances of quitting. While we have concentrated on individual treatments, this has to be in combination with individual governments strategically reviewing their public health policies and seeking to reduce the uptake of smoking by implementing policies such as health promotion, banning of smoking in public places, and applying tax duties appropriately.

References

Anthonisen NR, Connett JE, Kiley JP, *et al.* (1994). Effects of smoking intervention and the use of an inhaled anticholinergic bronchodilator on the rate of decline of FEV1. The Lung Health Study. *JAMA*, **272** (19), 1497–505.

Aveyard P and West R (2007). Managing smoking cessation. *British Medical Journal*, **335**, 37–41.

Bevins RA, Wilkinson JL, and Sanderson SD (2008). Vaccines to combat smoking. *Expert Opinion on Biological Therapy*, **8** (4), 379–83.

Buist AS, McBurnie MA, Vollmer WM *et al.* (2007). Bold Collaborative Research Group. International variation in the prevalence of COPD (the BOLD study): a population-based prevalence study. *Lancet*, **370** (9589), 741–50.

Cahill K and Ussher M (2007). Cannabinoid type 1 receptor antagonists (rimonabant) for smoking cessation. *Cochrane Database of Systematic Reviews*, **4**, CD005353.

Cahill K, Stead LF, and Lancaster T (2007). Nicotine receptor partial agonists for smoking cessation. *Cochrane Database of Systematic Reviews*, **1**, CD006103.

Fletcher C and Peto R (1977). The natural history of chronic airflow obstruction. *British Medical Journal*, **1** (6077), 1645–8.

Gartner CE, Hall WD, Vos T, *et al.* (2007). Assessment of Swedish snus for tobacco harm reduction: an epidemiological modelling study. *Lancet*, **369** (9578), 2010–4.

Hughes JR, Stead LF, and Lancaster T (2007). Antidepressants for smoking cessation. *Cochrane Database of Systematic Reviews*, **1**, CD000031.

Lancaster T and Stead L (2005a). Individual behavioural counselling for smoking cessation. *Cochrane Database of Systematic Reviews*, **2**, CD001292.

LancasterT and Stead LF (2005b). Self-help interventions for smoking cessation. *Cochrane Database of Systematic Reviews*, **3**, CD001118.

NICE Guideline (2007). Varenicline for smoking cessation. www.nice.org.uk/Guidance/TA123

Nides M (2008). Update on pharmacologic options for smoking cessation treatment. *The American Journal of Medicine*, **121** (4 Suppl 1), S20–31.

Parkes G, Greenhalgh T, Griffin M, and Dent R (2008). Effect on smoking quit rate of telling patients their lung age: the Step2quit randomised controlled trial. *British Medical Journal*, **336** (7644), 598–600.

Rice VH and Stead LF (2008). Nursing interventions for smoking cessation. *Cochrane Database of Systematic Reviews*, **1**, CD001188.

Richard Doll, Richard Peto, Jillian Boreham, and Isabelle Sutherland (2004). Mortality in relation to smoking: 50 years' observation on British male doctors. *British Medical Journal*, **328**, 1519.

Stead L and Lancaster T (2005). Group behaviour therapy programmes for smoking cessation. *Cochrane Database of Systematic Reviews*, **2**, CD001007.

Stead L, Bergson G, and Lancaster T (2008). Physician advice for smoking cessation. *Cochrane Database of Systematic Reviews*, **2**, CD000165.

Stead LF, Perera R, and Lancaster T (2006). Telephone counselling for smoking cessation. *Cochrane Database of Systematic Reviews*, **3**, CD002850.

Stead LF, Perera R, Bullen C, Mant D, and Lancaster T (2008). Nicotine replacement therapy for smoking cessation. *Cochrane Database of Systematic Reviews*, **1**, CD000146.

West R, McNeill A, and Raw M (2000). Smoking cessation guidelines for health professionals: an update. *Thorax*, **55**, 987–99.

Chapter 6

Chronic medical therapy and the GOLD guidelines

Miguel Carrera, Ernest Sala, and Alvar GN Agustí

Key points

- Active reduction of risk factors and bronchodilator treatment are central to the management of COPD.
- Regular use of long-acting bronchodilators (β_2-agonists and antimuscarinics) is more effective than short-acting bronchodilators in patients with persistent symptoms.
- Inhaled corticosteroids (ICS) combined with bronchodilators are indicated in patients with forced expiratory volume in 1s FEV_1 < 50% predicted and repeated exacerbations.
- Influenza vaccination is indicated for all COPD patients; while pneumococcal vaccine is recommended for COPD patients older than 65 years, and in those younger with FEV_1 < 40% predicted.
- Antibiotics should only be used for infectious exacerbations of COPD, while N-acetylcysteine only affects the frequency of exacerbations in patients off inhaled corticosteroids.
- Mucolytic agents, antitussives, and vasodilators are not recommended in stable COPD.
- All COPD patients benefit from exercise training programmes, while long-term oxygen therapy increases survival in COPD patients with chronic respiratory failure.

53

6.1 Introduction

Treatment of COPD has the following goals: (1) slow down the progression of the disease; (2) relieve symptoms; (3) improve health status; (4) improve exercise tolerance; (5) prevent and treat exacerbations and complications; and (6) reduce patient mortality. This chapter reviews: (1) the clinical pharmacology of the different drugs available to date for the treatment of COPD; and, (2) the indications and effectiveness of the different therapeutic options, according to the last update of the Global Initiative for Chronic Obstructive Lung Disease (GOLD 2007).

6.2 Pharmacological options

6.2.1 Bronchodilators

Bronchodilators constitute the cornerstone of the treatment of patients with COPD. Three types of bronchodilators are currently available: β_2-agonists, antimuscarinics, and theophylline. All of them relax airways smooth muscle but act through different pathways. β_2-agonists and antimuscarinics are the most effective. Administered by inhalation they achieve their greatest bronchodilator effect rapidly (Table 6.1) and have minimal secondary effects. There are different commercialized models of pressurized metered dose inhalers (MDI) and dry powder inhalers (DPI) that allow choice of devices for different patients. Occasionally, patients cannot use any of these devices correctly. In these cases, spacer devices are useful. If necessary bronchodilators can also be administered by means of nebulizers that do not require coordination by the patient. Spacer devices and nebulizers improve patient compliance but do not achieve greater bronchodilatation when compared to DPI and MDI devices used correctly. Theophylline is less effective as a bronchodilator than β_2-agonists and antimuscarinics and causes frequent side-effects (nausea, headache). However, it can be an addition to the other bronchodilators (β_2-agonists and antimuscarinics) if symptoms persist and are uncontrolled. Recent experimental evidence suggests that, at low doses, theophylline can improve the anti-inflammatory effects of steroids in COPD.

Table 6.1 Inhaled bronchodilators in the treatment of stable COPD				
	Start (mins)	Peak (mins)	Duration (hours)	Dosage (µg/hours)
Salbutamol (albuterol)	3–5	60–90	4–6	100–200/6–8
Terbutaline	3–5	60–90	4–6	400–500/6–8
Fenoterol	3–5	60–90	4–6	100–200/6–8
Formoterol	5	60–90	11–12	4.5–12/12
Salmeterol	45–60	120–240	11–12	25–50/12
Ipratropium bromide	5–15	60–120	6–8	20–40/6–8
Tiotropium	15	60–240	32	18/24

6.2.1.1 β_2-agonists

Salbutamol, terbutaline and fenoterol are short-acting β_2-agonists (SABAs). These drugs bind to β_2-adrenergic receptors, which are abundantly expressed in the airway smooth muscle and activate the enzyme adenylcyclase, which, in turn, increases the intracellular levels of cyclic adenosine monophosphate (cAMP), reduces the concentration of intracellular calcium, and produces bronchodilatation. β_2-Agonists therefore reduce airway resistance, air trapping, respiratory work, and dyspnoea, and improve health status. Their pharmacokinetic properties (rapid onset of action [3–5min] and relatively short duration of effect) makes SABAs particularly well suited as rescue medication (Table 6.1). At high doses SABAs may have undesired side effects such as tremour, tachycardia, and hypokalaemia.

Salmeterol and formoterol are long-acting β_2-agonists (LABAs). They have a slower onset of action than SABAs, but, in contrast, their effects last longer, which allows their administration every 12 hours (Table 6.1). Accordingly, they are mainly indicated for the maintenance treatment of COPD. Formoterol has a faster onset action than salmeterol (Table 6.1). This may allow its simultaneous use as maintenance and rescue medication. LABAs reduce symptoms more effectively than SABAs, improve health status, and reduce the number of exacerbations in patients with COPD. Different pharmaceutical companies are now developing LABAs with an even longer duration of action, which may allow once-daily use in the future.

6.2.1.2 Antimuscarinics

Through the release of acetylcholine, the parasympathetic nervous system can activate muscarinic receptors in exocrine glands and the central nervous system (M1 receptor), myocardium (M2 receptor), and airway smooth muscle (M3 receptor). The activation of these receptors reduce the intracellular cAMP concentration and, in the airways, produce bronchoconstriction. Antimuscarinics are drugs derived from atropine that have a greater affinity for muscarinic receptors than acetylcholine. Thus, they have the potential to block the action of acetylcholine and, in the airways, produce bronchodilatation. Administered by inhalation, less than 1% of these drugs reaches the systemic circulation, minimizing the undesired potential atropinic side effects (dryness of mouth, urinary retention).

Ipratropium bromide is a non-selective antimuscarinic bronchodilator (anticholinergic) that binds to M1, M2, and M3 receptors. Compared to SABAs, ipratropium bromide has a slower onset action, and a similar bronchodilator potency, and its effect lasts longer (Table 6.1). Tiotropium is a long-acting antimuscarinic bronchodilator (LAMA) which is 10-fold more potent than ipratropium (Table 6.1). Both ipratropium bromide and tiotropium bind to the same receptors, but tiotropium dissociates quickly from M2 receptors and very slowly from

M1 and M3. This explains its greater bronchodilatatory potency, long-lasting effects (35h), and relative selectivity. Tiotropium bromide reduces pulmonary hyperinflation, dyspnoea, and the number of exacerbations in COPD. Other long-acting antimuscarinics (such as aclidinium bromide) are currently being developed for treatment of COPD.

6.2.1.3 *Theophylline*

Theophylline is a non-selective phosphodiesterase inhibitor. It is a weak bronchodilator and a respiratory stimulant that improves diaphragmatic contractility. As a result, theophylline produces modest clinical and functional improvements. Furthermore, because its therapeutic range is narrow (plasma levels between 5 and 15 µg/mL) and its pharmacokinetics are influenced by multiple factors, its use is often associated with undesired side effects, including gastrointestinal (abdominal pain, nausea, and diarrhoea), cardiovascular (tachycardia, hypotension), and neurological (headache, insomnia) effects. The combination of its weak bronchodilator potency and frequent side effects makes theophylline a second-line drug in patients with COPD. It can be used, however, in patients with persistent symptoms despite optimal treatment with LABAs and LAMAs (see Section 6.2.1.4). In these patients, theophylline can be prescribed in addition to (never instead of) regular therapy. However, there is some in vitro evidence that at much lower doses than used clinically (when bronchodilation is the goal), theophylline activates the activity of histone deacetylase and, by doing so, enhances the anti-inflammatory effects of steroids. These in vitro observations need to be translated into the clinical arena before specific practical recommendations can be made.

6.2.1.4 *Combined bronchodilator therapy*

Patients whose symptoms are not controlled by one bronchodilator alone can benefit from a combination of drugs that act by different mechanisms. Ipratropium bromide and SABAs administered jointly produce greater bronchodilatation than each one separately. The combination of LABAs and LAMA also has an additive effect. Theophylline can be used when symptoms persist despite the use of two long-acting bronchodilators.

6.2.2 **Corticosteroids**

6.2.2.1 *Inhaled corticosteroids*

According to GOLD, COPD is characterized by airflow limitation that in not fully reversible, usually progressive, and associated with an abnormal inflammatory response of the lung to noxious particles or gases. Inhaled corticosteroids (e.g. beclometasone, budesonide, fluticasone) appear to reduce inflammation in COPD. In patients with severe COPD and persistent symptoms despite bronchodilator treatment, inhaled corticosteroids contribute to clinical control and reduce the number of exacerbations.

6.2.2.2 *Systemic corticosteroids*

Systemic corticosteroids (oral or intravenous) are not indicated for the maintenance treatment of COPD because of their significant side effects (osteoporosis, muscle atrophy, cataracts, hypertension). They are used, however, for the treatment of acute exacerbations. Yet, the clinical response to acute treatment with these drugs does not predict benefit in long term nor the response to inhaled corticosteroids. Exceptionally, in patients with very severe disease, uncontrolled symptoms, and frequent exacerbations despite maximal inhaled therapy (plus theophylline), systemic steroids can be prescribed at the minimal doses possible (if possible every 48h).

6.2.3 Combination therapy

In patients with FEV1 < 60% predicted, the combination of salmeterol and fluticasone improves lung function, symptoms, health status, number of exacerbations, and, potentially, survival. Adding tiotropium (triple combination) provides additional benefit on lung function, degree of dyspnoea, and health status, although it does not reduce the number or severity of exacerbations.

6.2.4 Other drugs

In general, mucolytics, expectorants, and antitussives have not demonstrated any benefit in COPD patients. *N*-acetylcysteine is a mucolytic and antioxidant that seems to reduce the frequency of exacerbations in those patients not treated with inhaled corticosteroids. At present, the GOLD guidelines do not recommend any of these drugs in COPD. There is no evidence to support the use of antibiotics in the chronic management of COPD, although they may be indicated during the course of an infective exacerbation of the disease.

6.2.5 Vaccines

Influenza vaccines containing killed or inactivated virus reduce severe exacerbations and death in patients with COPD by 50% and should be prescribed in all COPD patients. The pneumococcal vaccine is recommended for patients with COPD $\geq$ 65yrs. In addition, this vaccine has been shown to reduce the incidence of pneumonia in COPD patients younger than 65yrs with a FEV_1 < 40% predicted. At present, there is no data that supports the routine use of an anti-haemophilus vaccination.

6.3 Therapeutic strategy of clinically stable COPD

GOLD grades the severity of COPD according to the degree of airflow limitation (determined post-bronchodilatation). It should be noted that using this parameter alone is probably insufficient because airflow obstruction does not describe the different pulmonary and extra-pulmonary domains of the disease. However, current treatment recommendations are mainly based on this classification (Figure 6.1).

Irrespective of airflow obstruction, smoking cessation, regular physical activity, and annual influenza, vaccination should be recommended in all COPD. Furthermore, education in the general aspects of the disease, as well as in the correct use of inhalers, helps patients to understand and accept their disease better, improves treatment compliance, and contributes to better health status.

SABAs or ipratropium bromide can be used on demand in patients with mild COPD (FEV1 ≥ 80% predicted; Stage I) and occasional symptoms. In contrast, patients with persistent symptoms, generally associated with moderate airflow obstruction (FEV$_1$ between 50 and 80% predicted; Stage II), should be treated regularly with long-acting bronchodilators (LABAs or LAMAs). If this strategy does not control symptoms adequately, a combination of one LABA and one LAMA has been shown to be more effective than each one separately.

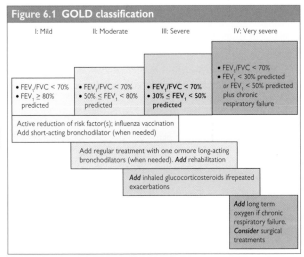

Figure 6.1 GOLD classification

I: Mild	II: Moderate	III: Severe	IV: Very severe
• FEV$_1$/FVC < 70% • FEV$_1$ ≥ 80% predicted	• FEV$_1$/FVC < 70% • 50% ≤ FEV$_1$ < 80% predicted	• **FEV$_1$/FVC < 70%** • **30% ≤ FEV$_1$ < 50% predicted**	• FEV$_1$/FVC < 70% • FEV$_1$ < 30% predicted or FEV$_1$ < 50% predicted plus chronic respiratory failure

Active reduction of risk factor(s); influenza vaccination
Add short-acting bronchodilator (when needed)

Add regular treatment with one ormore long-acting bronchodilators (when needed). **Add** rehabilitation

Add inhaled glucocorticosteroids ifrepeated exacerbations

Add long term oxygen if chronic respiratory failure. **Consider** surgical treatments

In severe or very severe COPD (FEV_1 between 50 and 30% predicted; and <30% predicted; Stage III and IV respectively), GOLD recommends the addition of inhaled corticosteroids to long-acting bronchodilators in subjects with repeated exacerbations. The recently published TORCH study did not find a statistically significant effect of inhaled corticosteroids on mortality ($p = 0.052$) but the observed reduction in the relative risk of death (17.5%) is likely to be clinically significant. Short-acting bronchodilators on demand can be prescribed on top of chronic therapy if necessary. In patients with uncontrolled symptoms despite maximal inhaled therapy, theophylline may be prescribed too.

In general, available drugs are very effective. The main reasons for treatment failure are poor inhaler technique (supporting the importance of education in each visit in the clinic) and, perhaps, an excessive number of inhalers prescribed (an argument supporting the use of combination therapy if indicated).

Non-pharmacological therapeutic alternatives are also important in these patients, and include pulmonary rehabilitation (indicated in patients with moderate COPD and persistent symptoms despite appropriate drug treatment) and nutritional support if needed. Domiciliary oxygen therapy and surgical options (including lung volume reduction surgery and lung transplant) should be taken into account in the more severe patients. These alternatives are discussed at length in other companion chapters.

Key reference

National Institute for Health (NIH), National Heart Lung and Blood Institute of the USA (NHLBI), and the World Health Organization (WHO), Global Initiative for Chronic Obstructive Lung Disease (GOLD): Global strategy for the diagnosis, management, and prevention of COPD. http://www.goldcopd.org, Updated in 2007.

References

Aaron SD, Vandemheen KL, Fergusson D, et al.; Canadian Thoracic Society/ Canadian Respiratory Clinical Research Consortium (2007). Tiotropium in combination with placebo, salmeterol, or fluticasone-salmeterol for treatment of chronic obstructive pulmonary disease: a randomized trial. Annals of Internal Medicine, 146, 545–55.

Agusti AG (2005). COPD, a multicomponent disease: implications for management. Respiratory Medicine, 99, 670–82.

Alfageme I, Vazquez R, Reyes N, et al. (2006). Clinical efficacy of anti-pneumococcal vaccination in patients with COPD. Thorax, 61, 189–95.

Barnes PJ (2006). The pharmacological properties of tiotropium. Chest, 117, 63S–6S.

Burge PS, Calverley PM, Jones PW, Spencer S, Anderson JA, and Maslen TK (2000). Randomised, double blind, placebo controlled study of fluticasone propionate in patients with moderate to severe chronic obstructive pulmonary disease: the ISOLDE trial. *British Medical Journal*, **320**, 1297–303.

Campbell M, Eliraz A, Johansson G, *et al.* (2005). Formoterol for maintenance and as-needed treatment of chronic obstructive pulmonary disease. *Respiratory Medicine*, **99**, 1511–20.

Calverley P, Pauwels R, Vestbo J, *et al.*; TRial of Inhaled STeroids ANd long-acting beta2 agonists study group (2003). Combined salmeterol and fluticasone in the treatment of chronic obstructive pulmonary disease: a randomised controlled trial. *Lancet*, **361**, 449–56.

Calverley PM, Anderson JA, Celli B, *et al.*; TORCH investigators (2007). Salmeterol and fluticasone propionate and survival in chronic obstructive pulmonary disease. *The New England Journal of Medicine*, **356**, 775–89.

Celli BR and MacNee W (2004). Standards for the diagnosis and treatment of patients with COPD: a summary of the ATS/ERS position paper. *The European Respiratory Journal*, 23, 932–46.

Decramer M, Rutten-van Mölken M, Dekhuijzen PN, *et al.* (2005). Effects of N-acetylcysteine on outcomes in chronic obstructive pulmonary disease (Bronchitis Randomized on NAC Cost-Utility Study, BRONCUS): a randomised placebo-controlled trial. *Lancet*, **365**, 1552–60.

Dusser D, Bravo ML, and Iacono P (2006). The effect of tiotropium on exacerbations and airflow in patients with COPD. *The European Respiratory Journal*, **27**, 547–55.

Hanania NA and Donohue JF (2007). Pharmacologic interventions in chronic obstructive pulmonary disease: bronchodilators. *Proceedings of the American Thoracic Society*, **4**, 526–34.

Lavorini F, Magnan A, Christophe Dubus J, *et al.* (2008). Effect of incorrect use of dry powder inhalers on management of patients with asthma and COPD. *Respiratory Medicine*, **102**, 593–604.

Stockley RA, Chopra N, and Rice L. (2006). Addition of salmeterol to existing treatment in patients with COPD: a 12 month study. *Thorax*, **61**, 122–28.

van Noord JA, Aumann JL, Janssens E, *et al.* (2005). Comparison of tiotropium once daily, formoterol twice daily and both combined once daily in patients with COPD. *The European Respiratory Journal*, **26**, 214–22.

Wedzicha JA, Calverley PM, Seemungal TA, Hagan G, Ansari Z, and Stockley RA (2008). The prevention of chronic obstructive pulmonary disease exacerbations by salmeterol/fluticasone propionate or tiotropium bromide. *American Journal of Respiratory and Critical Care Medicine*, **177**, 19–26.

Wilt TJ, Niewoehner D, Macdonald R, and Kane RL (2007). Management of stable chronic obstructive pulmonary disease: a systematic review for a clinical practice guideline. *Annals of Internal Medicine*, **147**, 639–53.

Chapter 7

Management of acute exacerbations including non-invasive and invasive ventilation

Clare L.K. Ross, Onn Min Kon, and William L.G. Oldfield

Key points

- An exacerbation of chronic obstructive pulmonary disease (COPD) is a sustained worsening of a patient's symptoms from their usual stable state, which is beyond normal day-to-day variations, and is acute in onset.
- Oxygen supplementation should be given in a controlled manner to maintain adequate levels of oxygenation. If hypercapnia and a respiratory acidosis develop or worsen, ventilatory support should be considered.
- Medical management consists of bronchodilators, corticosteroids, and, in some situations, antibiotics. Adequate hydration and nutrition should also be provided.
- Non-invasive ventilation (NIV) should be instituted, in addition to medical management, in patients with acute hypercapnic respiratory failure with an associated respiratory acidosis (pH < 7.35).
- Patients can often be managed in a Hospital-at-Home (HaH) scheme after careful consideration of symptom severity, co-morbidities, baseline function, and home situation.

7.1 Medical management and acute exacerbations

7.1.1 Definition

An exacerbation of COPD is a sustained worsening of a patient's symptoms from their usual stable state, which is beyond normal day-to-day variations, and is acute in onset.

7.1.2 Presentation

The most frequently reported symptoms are worsening breathlessness, wheeze, cough, increased sputum production, and a change in sputum colour or purulence. Patients may also present with less specific symptoms such as confusion, impaired consciousness, fluid retention, and increased fatigue. Common triggers include bacterial infections (typically *H. influenzae*, *S. pneumoniae*, *M. catarrhalis*, *S. aureus*, or *P. aeruginosa*), viral infections (typically rhinoviruses, influenza, parainfluenza, coronavirus, adenovirus, or respiratory syncitial virus), or common pollutants such as sulphur dioxide. Alternative and/or additional diagnoses must be considered, for example pneumonia, thromboembolism, pneumothorax, and left ventricular failure.

7.1.3 Initial examination and investigations

Good history taking is vital. It is important to establish the patient's normal level of functioning, their usual medications and allergies, and co-morbidities; quantify any previous hospital admissions with exacerbations; and determine whether intubation or non-invasive ventilation (NIV) is appropriate. Previous lung function results, arterial blood gas (ABG) tensions, and imaging can be very useful.

Examination must assess the degree of respiratory distress (respiratory rate [RR], the use of accessory muscles, and paradoxical chest wall movements). It is important to look for signs of *cor pulmonale* such as peripheral oedema, and evidence of hypoxia or hypercapnia. The following investigations should be performed:

- **CXR**: to look for alternative or co-existing pathology
- **ABG**: to quantify the degree of respiratory failure and guide oxygen therapy (it is vital to record the inspired oxygen concentration [FiO_2] at the time the ABG is taken)
- **ECG**: to look for alternative or co-existing pathology
- **FBC**: to look for leukocytosis or secondary polycythaemia
- **U&E**: to look for evidence of dehydration or renal impairment and assess K^+ levels which can be affected by bronchodilator and corticosteroid treatment
- **LFTs**: to look for derangement if an atypical pneumonia is considered

- **Glucose**: to provide a baseline prior to commencing steroid therapy, especially if there is a history of diabetes
- **Theophylline level**: if the patient takes theophylline at home
- **Sputum sample**: for microscopy, culture and sensitivities
- **Blood cultures**: if the patient is pyrexial.

7.1.4 Assessment of severity and need for hospital admission

Several options exist when deciding where to manage a patient. If the exacerbation is mild they can be discharged on oral and inhaled medication. If the exacerbation is more severe, hospital-based treatment is indicated. This can be provided either by way of hospital admission (with or without the subsequent provision of an early assisted discharge) or by way of the 'Hospital-at-Home' (HaH) scheme. The latter is a specific form of intermediate care whereby healthcare professionals provide treatment for a patient in their own home, which would otherwise require hospital admission. The multidisciplinary team required to operate this scheme comprises of doctors, nurses, physiotherapists, occupational therapists, and generic health care workers. If a patient is deemed suitable for HaH, a care package is prescribed which includes steroids, nebulized bronchodilators, antibiotics if indicated, and oxygen if necessary. Hospitals which provide a HaH scheme will have their own guidelines and staff responsible for initiating the process. The decision whether to treat at home or to admit the patient to hospital must be based on several factors, namely the severity of the patient's condition, their home situation, their wishes, and their compliance with treatment. Some criteria for hospital admission are detailed in Table 7.1.

7.1.5 Management

7.1.5.1 Oxygen

Oxygen supplementation should be given to maintain adequate levels of oxygenation. Maintaining levels initially between 88 and 92% aims to do this without precipitating or worsening hypercapnia and thus a

Table 7.1 Criteria for hospital admission

- PaO_2 <7kPa
- Respiratory acidosis
- Radiological evidence of pneumonia
- Severe breathlessness
- Worsening peripheral oedema
- Established home oxygen
- Confusion or impaired consciousness
- Immobility and inability to cope at home
- Multiple co-morbidities
- Rapid-onset exacerbations

respiratory acidosis (in some COPD patients respiratory drive depends on their degree of hypoxia rather than the usual dependence on hypercapnia). Controlled oxygen therapy via a Venturi mask is the preferred mode of delivery, starting with 24% or 28% oxygen. ABG analysis should be performed as early as possible in order to guide further oxygen supplementation and assess the need for ventilation. Any change in oxygen therapy should be followed by repeat ABG analysis 30 to 60 min later. Patients with acute type 2 respiratory failure and a respiratory acidosis who fail to respond to maximal medical therapy should be considered for ventilatory support—see Section 7.2.

7.1.5.2 *Drugs*

Bronchodilators are required, usually in the form of nebulized therapy, to ensure maximal drug delivery. Examples include salbutamol 2.5–5mg every 2 to 4h (as well as on a PRN basis), and ipratropium bromide 500mcg every 6h. These should be driven by compressed air rather than oxygen if there is a tendency for the patient to become hypercapnic. The patient's usual short-acting inhaled therapy is stopped temporarily whilst on nebulized therapy (their inhaled long-acting therapy should continue). Nebulizers can also be given to patients entering the HaH scheme. Once the patient's condition improves, nebulizers should be discontinued in favour of inhaled bronchodilators. It is important to check the patient's technique—the addition of a spacer device can improve drug delivery significantly. Side effects related to bronchodilator therapy include tachycardia, hypokalaemia, and, in the case of antimuscarinic agents, pupillary dilatation.

Oral corticosteroids (i.e. prednisolone 30mg daily for 7 to 14 days) should be considered in all patients. With short courses of prednisolone a reducing-dose regimen is not necessary; however, if the patient's condition remains poor, a slower tailing-off of steroid therapy may be indicated. In patients requiring multiple courses of oral steroids, osteoporosis should be considered. DEXA scanning may be indicated in addition to prophylactic medication. The patients' usual inhaled steroid should be continued during an acute exacerbation.

Antibiotics should not be used routinely in all exacerbations of COPD. They are indicated when there is a combination of increased sputum volume, increased sputum purulence, or increased shortness of breath. Antibiotic choice is usually dictated by individual hospital guidelines and patient allergies but should generally be with an amin-openicillin, a macrolide, or a tetracycline. As in all situations where antibiotics are indicated, the first dose should be given on admission after acquisition of the relevant cultures. Resistant strains of some common pathogens are now emerging and antibiotic therapy should be tailored towards a specific sensitive pathogen if at all possible, once sensitivities are acquired.

Theophylline is a second-line drug which can be considered if there has been an inadequate response to usual medical therapy and in hypercapnic respiratory failure. Care should be taken in view of the potential for toxicity and drug interactions. Levels should be monitored within the first 24h of treatment. The loading dose should be omitted if the patient is already established on theophylline and has levels in the therapeutic range. Common side effects are nausea, tachycardia, and tremor.

Respiratory stimulants such as doxapram are no longer routinely recommended in the management of acute COPD exacerbations.

7.1.5.3 *Hydration and nutrition*

Patients with an exacerbation are likely to have increased insensible fluid losses. Intravenous fluids are required in a dehydrated patient. Those on NIV are particularly at risk since the mask will prevent frequent oral intake of fluid. It is important to ensure the patient is receiving adequate nutrition, and dietetic input may be helpful.

7.1.5.4 *Physiotherapy*

Physiotherapy is a vital part of medical management. Sputum clearance is often a problem in patients with acute exacerbations. Positive expiratory pressure masks can be helpful in some patients.

7.1.6 Discharge planning

Prior to discharge patients should be established on appropriate long-term medication. Inhaler technique should be checked. All patients should have spirometry and ABG analysis performed prior to discharge. If there is concern about a patient's ability to manage at home, a formal assessment should be performed. Patients should be given information about their condition and medications, and a management plan for guidance in the event of deterioration. Patients should be followed up in a chest clinic, and those with pneumonia should have a repeat CXR at 4–6 weeks to ensure resolution.

7.2 Non-invasive ventilation (NIV)

7.2.1 Introduction to NIV

Non-invasive positive pressure ventilation (NIV or NIPPV) is the delivery of mechanically assisted breaths or mechanically generated breaths without placement of an invasive artificial airway such as an endotracheal tube. Ventilation is usually delivered via a tight-fitting face or nasal mask with alternatives including helmets or nasal pillows.

NIV improves alveolar ventilation, reduces the work of breathing, and reduces morbidity and mortality in acute respiratory failure, complicating COPD. It is associated with a shorter length of hospital stay and a reduction in the need for invasive ventilation. NIV allows for intermittent ventilatory support, encouraging normal eating and drinking, communication, physiotherapy sessions, and provision of nebulized medication.

Continuous positive airway pressure (CPAP) is often included in discussions regarding NIV. Strictly speaking CPAP is not a form of ventilatory support in that it does not provide assistance during inspiration. It aims to improve oxygenation rather than ventilation by improving alveolar recruitment and increasing functional residual capacity and thus should not be instituted when hypercapnia is the underlying concern. CPAP is thus used in type 1 respiratory failure, and NIV is used in type 2 respiratory failure. The term 'BiPAP' refers to a specific Bi-level ventilator manufactured by the Respironics Corporation. This machine has been used in some NIV trials and the term 'BiPAP' is often used interchangeably with NIV.

The principles of treating type 2 respiratory failure rely on reducing the pCO_2 (which is inversely proportional to a patient's minute ventilation [tidal volume x RR]) and increasing the pO_2 (which is proportional to the mean airway pressure and FiO_2). NIV, that is Bi-level ventilation, uses two different pressures, an inspiratory positive airway pressure (IPAP) and an expiratory positive airway pressure (EPAP). The EPAP is sometimes referred to as the positive-end expiratory pressure (PEEP). IPAP assists inspiration, thus increasing tidal volume and facilitating CO_2 removal. EPAP eliminates exhaled air through the exhalation port, encourages lung recruitment (increasing the functional residual capacity and the surface area for gas exchange), stents open the upper airway, and overcomes the intrinsic PEEP (auto-PEEP) present in many patients with COPD. Both components of the cycle reduce the work of breathing.

7.2.2 Indications for acute NIV

NIV should be instituted in addition to medical management in all COPD patients with acute (or acute-on-chronic) type 2 respiratory failure with a respiratory acidosis (pH 7.25–7.35, H^+ 45–56nmol/L) who fail to respond to maximal medical therapy (Table 7.2). ABG tensions should therefore be measured in all individuals with breathlessness of sufficient severity to warrant admission to hospital. It is important to interpret the ABGs in the light of the FiO_2 required to maintain a paO_2 of ≥8kPa. Many patients may improve rapidly with maximal medical therapy and appropriate supplemental oxygen, as detailed above. A repeat ABG should therefore be taken after a short interval to establish whether NIV is indicated. NIV may be undertaken as a therapeutic trial with a view to tracheal intubation if NIV fails, or conversely, NIV may be the ceiling of treatment for patients who are poor candidates for tracheal intubation. It is therefore vital that a decision regarding tracheal intubation. It is therefore

Table 7.2 Selection criteria for NIV (GOLD, 2007)

- Moderate to severe dyspnoea with use of accessory muscles and paradoxical abdominal movement
- Respiratory frequency >25 beats/min
- Moderate to severe acidosis pH ≤7.35 and/or hypercapnoea $PaCO_2$ >6.0kPa.

Table 7.3 Contraindications to NIV (* not absolute)

- Inability to maintain own airway*
- Facial trauma/burns
- Vomiting
- Fixed upper airway obstruction
- Bronchial ± pleural fistula
- High risk of aspiration
- Recent facial/upper airway/upper gastrointestinal surgery*
- Copious respiratory secretions*
- Bowel obstruction*
- Life-threatening hypoxaemia*
- Severe co-morbidity*
- Suspected/confirmed pneumothorax without an intercostal drain *in situ**
- Haemodynamic instability*
- Focal consolidation on CXR*
- Impaired consciousness*
- Confusion/agitation*.

vital that a decision regarding intubation is made when a patient is first started on NIV. This should not be used instead of tracheal intubation if the latter is clearly more appropriate.

7.2.3 Contraindications to NIV

Numerous contraindications to NIV exist, as detailed in Table 7.3. These must be interpreted in the clinical setting. NIV can still be used in certain situations (*) provided a clear plan is in place if NIV fails, that is a decision to insert an endotracheal tube or a decision that NIV is the 'ceiling' of treatment. Close monitoring is even more important if NIV is used in any of these situations.

7.2.4 Set-up of equipment

7.2.4.1 *Machine*

Numerous different machines exist which can provide NIV. Most machines use bi-level pressure support (whereby the IPAP is fixed at a set level above EPAP), but volume-controlled non-invasive ventilators also exist (whereby the desired tidal volume to be delivered is set and the inspiratory pressure varies as required). Pressure-controlled

Table 7.4 Modes of NIV	
Spontaneous	Patient initiates all breaths. These breaths are detected by the machine trigger and supported with supplemental pressure.
Spontaneous timed	Patients can still initiate breaths, which are then supported, but a back-up rate of machine-delivered breaths is also set. For example, the back-up rate may be set to 5 breaths per minute less than the patient's spontaneous rate. This is the most appropriate setting for NIV.
Timed	This fully ventilates those patients making no respiratory effort and is therefore generally an inappropriate mode for NIV.

machines are more common. The precise machine will vary between hospitals, and it is important to familiarize yourself with the machines available.

7.2.4.2 *Mode*
Three options exist (see Table 7.4).

7.2.4.3 *Mask*
Numerous different interfaces exist, including nasal masks, face masks which cover the nose and mouth, face masks which cover the entire face, nasal plugs, and even helmets. The initial mask of choice should be a face mask which covers the patient's nose and mouth. These generally come in three different sizes, and it is important to determine the most appropriate size for the patient to ensure a tight seal and achieve maximal comfort. Often the packaging of the masks has a template cut-out which can be used as an aid to choose the correct size.

Obtain consent and invest time in explaining to the patient what NIV is and how their condition will be managed. This will increase the likelihood of success. Hold the mask initially over the patients face, applying light pressure. When the patient is comfortable apply the head straps and tighten to eliminate leaks.

7.2.4.4 *Settings*
Suggested initial settings are an IPAP of 12cm H_2O (8cm H_2O over EPAP), an EPAP of 4cm H_2O and 2L/min of supplemental oxygen, aiming for SpO_2 of 88–92%. NIV should be continuous for the first 24h, allowing breaks only for meals, physiotherapy, and nebulizers (these can be given via a T-piece fitted into the NIV circuit if the equipment is available).

7.2.5 Monitoring
Patients requiring NIV should be cared for in a specialist area. This may be a respiratory ward staffed by nurses familiar with NIV, or a high-dependency or intensive care unit.

Observations should include blood pressure, heart rate, RR, and oxygen saturations. The latter should be monitored continuously. Clinical examination should be performed at regular intervals and include measurement of RR, observation of the use of accessory muscles of respiration, paradoxical movements of the chest wall, and coordination of respiratory effort with the ventilator. Auscultation should be performed. Patient comfort and mental state should be regularly assessed.

Investigations should include an ABG at 1h and then again at approximately 4–6h based on initial findings. Any changes in NIV settings should be followed by a repeat ABG at 30–60min. If there has been no improvement after 4–6h, NIV is unlikely to be successful and discontinuation of NIV should be considered with a view to endotracheal intubation or palliation. A chest X-ray (CXR) should be performed in the event of any acute deterioration, looking for evidence of a pneumothorax or aspiration.

Several factors should be taken into account when deciding if a patient is an appropriate candidate for invasive ventilation and intensive care. These include the patient's age, baseline FEV_1, functional status, BMI, their requirement for oxygen when stable, co-morbidities, and previous admissions to intensive care units.

7.2.6 Troubleshooting

See Table 7.5.

7.2.7 Weaning from NIV

Weaning can be commenced after 24h if the patient is improving. There are various ways of doing this, the simplest being increasing the duration of time the patient is not wearing the mask. Initially, this should be for meal times, then for longer daytime periods, and then finally overnight also.

7.3 Invasive mechanical ventilation (IMV)

Full active intervention during acute exacerbations of COPD is recommended, as mortality from COPD patients with respiratory failure is lower than mortality from other causes. IMV is more effective when there is likely to be reversibility of the acute cause. The patient's wishes should be paramount and the hazards of IMV considered.

7.3.1 Indications for IMV (GOLD, 2007)

- Unable to tolerate or respond to NIV
- Severe dyspnoea with use of accessory muscles and paradoxical abdominal movement
- Respiratory frequency >35/min
- Life-threatening hypoxaemia

Table 7.5 Troubleshooting guide	
Problem encountered	Actions to consider
Inadequate ventilatory support (persisting acidosis/ high CO_2)	Check for leaks Check expiratory port is not blocked Clinical re-evaluation Wean FiO_2 if SpO_2 is >94% Increase IPAP in increments of 2–4cm H_2O and repeat ABG after 30–60min. Ensure optimal additional medical management.
Persisting hypoxia	Check for leaks Clinical re-evaluation Increase EPAP in increments of 2cm H_2O (and IPAP by the same amount) and repeat ABG after 30–60min Increase FiO_2 and repeat ABG after 30–60min Ensure optimal additional medical management
Leak from mask	Adjust straps Consider pressure dressing to cheeks/nose
Nasal and forehead damage	Apply padded dressing
Swallowing air into stomach	Insert NG tube
Eye irritation	Adjust mask fitting
Asynchrony	Consider different mode or machine. Discuss with senior; it may be necessary to adjust the pressure rise time or the inspiratory trigger.

- Severe acidosis pH <7.25 and /or hypercapnoea $PaCO_2$ >8.0kPa
- Respiratory arrest
- Somnolence
- Cardiovascular complications
- Other complications: metabolic abnormalities, sepsis, pneumonia, pulmonary embolism, barotraumas, massive pleural effusion.

When there is difficulty weaning from IMV, NIV can be considered.

Key reference

National Institute for Health (NIH), National Heart Lung and Blood Institute of the USA (NHLBI), and the World Health Organization (WHO), Global Initiative for Chronic Obstructive Lung Disease (GOLD): Global strategy for the diagnosis, management, and prevention of COPD. http://www.goldcopd.org, Updated in 2007.

References

NICE (2004). Chronic obstructive pulmonary disease—management of chronic obstructive pulmonary disease in adults in primary care and secondary care. www.nice.org.uk/guidance/CG12

British Thoracic Society (2007). Intermediate care—Hospital-at-Home in chronic obstructive pulmonary disease: British Thoracic Society guideline. *Thorax*, **62**, 200–10.

NICE (2004). Management of exacerbations of COPD. *Thorax*, **59**, 131–56.

British Thoracic Society Standards of Care Committee (2002). Non-invasive ventilation in acute respiratory failure. *Thorax*, **57**, 192–211.

Quon BS, Gan WQ, and Sin DD (2008). Contemporary management of acute exacerbations of COPD: a systematic review and metaanalysis. *Chest*, **133** (3), 756–66.

Chapter 8

Pulmonary rehabilitation

Thierry Troosters and Marc Decramer

Key points

- Pulmonary rehabilitation is an evidence-based therapy for patients with COPD who have impaired health-related quality of life, reduced exercise tolerance, reduced participation in activities of daily life, or excessive utilization of health care recourses, despite optimal medication.
- Programs are individually tailored, but exercise training is the cornerstone of the program.
- The exercise training program should adhere to exercise training guidelines for elderly, but specific modification may be needed based on the exercise limitation of the individual patient.
- Other relevant disciplines involved in the rehabilitation process of selected patients are nurses, nutritional specialists, occupational therapists, and social workers.
- Although the ultimate goal of pulmonary rehabilitation is to enhance physical activity, more research is needed to investigate how the benefits of pulmonary rehabilitation may spin off to enhanced physical activity.

8.1 Introduction

The evidence base for pulmonary rehabilitation is now so compelling that it is now considered a therapy which should be offered to patients with lung diseases who are symptomatic and have reduced activities of daily living, despite optimal medical therapy (Table 8.1). Unlike most drugs, pulmonary rehabilitation does not target the lungs directly; rather it aims at reversing or stabilizing the extra-pulmonary effects of lung diseases.

These extra-pulmonary effects of COPD do impact on the morbidity and the mortality of the disease. For example, skeletal muscle weakness and exercise intolerance are independent predictors of poor survival in patients with COPD. In addition, skeletal muscle weakness is an important driver of utilization of health care recourses. In the context of pulmonary rehabilitation it is also important to recognize non-physiological extra-pulmonary consequences of chronic lung disease.

Depression, for example, is very prevalent in stable patients, and it is a factor significantly related to adverse outcome of COPD, particularly after acute exacerbations. These exacerbations are important events which drive disease progression in COPD. Physical activity levels are reduced in patients suffering from exacerbations, and functional exercise capacity and health-related quality of life decline more rapidly in patients with frequent exacerbations.

Any therapy which improves muscle function and exercise tolerance, improves the physiological and non-physiological extra-pulmonary consequences of the disease, and reduces the severity of the number of exacerbations may impact successfully on the overall progression of COPD morbidity and perhaps even mortality. Pulmonary rehabilitation does enhance symptoms, improves health-related quality of life, enhances exercise tolerance and skeletal muscle function, and may reduce the severity of acute exacerbations.

Table 8.1 An overview of the effects of pulmonary rehabilitation as reported in evidence-based practice guidelines

Effect	Evidence grade	Size of effect
Improvement of dyspnoea	1A	CRDQ-Dys: 1.06 [0.85–1.26] points
Improvement of HRQoL	1A	SGRQ total: −6.11 [−8.98–3.24]%
Reduction in hospital days and utilization of health care recourses	2B	
Survival	None provided	
Psychosocial benefits (self-efficacy with exercise, cognitive function, anxiety, depression,)	2B	
Exercise tolerance Peak work rate 6MWD Whole-body endurance	1A	8W [3–13W] + 18 [IQR 13–24]% baseline 48m [32–65m] +34m if <28 sess, 50m if >28 sess. +87% of baseline

Evidence grading 1A: strong recommendation, 2B: Weak recommendation.
CRDQ-Dys: dyspnoea subscale of the chronic respiratory disease questionnaire,
SGRQ: Saint George's Respiratory Questionnaire; 6MWD: six-minute walking distance.

8.2 **General design of pulmonary rehabilitation programs**

In order to be successful, pulmonary rehabilitation is typically designed as a comprehensive intervention offered by a team of health care providers over a substantial period of time.

Typically rehabilitation programs are carried out for 6 weeks to 6 months, with longer programs yielding greater effects.

Patients participate in an individualized tailored program, which takes into account the complexity of the presenting patient.

Exercise training is the cornerstone of such a program, but several other interventions may complement the program in order to maximize its effectiveness.

Typical teams of health care providers, delivering pulmonary rehabilitation programs, include a chest physician, physiotherapists, a nurse specialist, an occupational therapist, a psychologist, a nutritional specialist, and a social worker.

Sometimes the general practitioner of the patients as well as the health care providers involved in the home care, pharmacists, and case managers may be part of the rehabilitation team.

Clearly the patient and his or her family should be active partners in the rehabilitation efforts.

8.3 **Screening and intake procedure**

Across centres there is significant variability in the intake procedure. There is only one constant: far too little patients are enrolled in rehabilitation. Recent estimates suggest that less than only 2% of patients of COPD patients have access to rehabilitation programs and are enrolled. Efforts should be made to encourage patients to participate in rehabilitation and sufficient programs should be available.

According to the definition of the American Thoracic Society and the European Respiratory Society, pulmonary rehabilitation is aiming at reducing symptoms, optimizing function, increasing participation, and reducing health care cost through stabilizing or reversing the systemic consequences of the disease. Hence, theoretically, patients with an indication for rehabilitation are those suffering from extrapulmonary consequences. This definition is, however, not very practical as the systemic consequences that can be targeted by pulmonary rehabilitation are not defined.

A more practical approach to identifying candidates for rehabilitation and guide the assessment of patients before enrolment in rehabilitation may be to select patients who are optimally pharmacologically treated but still present with one of the following:
• Disabling symptoms due to deconditioning

- Skeletal or respiratory muscle weakness
- Poor health-related quality of life
- Repeated exacerbations or inefficient use of available recourses
- Depressed mood status
- Malnutrition (obesity of cachexia)
- Poor coping with the symptoms of their disease.

This allows to set up active screening for rehabilitation programs, which typically includes assessment of exercise tolerance, skeletal and respiratory muscle force, nutritional status, symptoms, health-related quality of life, and capability of self-management. It is important to notice that age and lung function impairment are not exclusion criteria for exercise training. Importantly, although most research has been carried out in patients with stable COPD, patients after acute exacerbations appear to be particularly good candidates for pulmonary rehabilitation. Enrolment in a rehabilitation program after an acute exacerbation reduces the risk for relapse and may even improve survival.

Depending on the individual problems the program can be designed across a range of complexities. Programs can be as simple as an intervention consisting of exercise training in the home setting in patients with uncomplicated COPD or as complex as an inpatient program in a mechanically ventilated patient. On the basis of proper assessment the individual program, its setting, and components can be designed, taking into account the available recourses in a given region, current best practice, and evidence. Several guidelines may help those setting up pulmonary rehabilitation facilities to structure their program.

8.4 Setting of pulmonary rehabilitation

The setting of the rehabilitation program is an important point for consideration. Programs have been successfully set up in a primary care (home) setting, as an outpatient program in a rehabilitation centre or in the community or as an inpatient program. Clearly each of these programs has advantages and disadvantages. One of the most important problems of home-based programs is the limited staff and equipment, which makes it difficult to deal with more severe patients. When programs are carried out in the home setting but by the same staff, effects may be comparable to outpatient programs. The most important problem of outpatient programs is the transportation to the centre. Inpatient programs are costly and should be restricted to those patients with very limited mobility. Ideally a reference rehabilitation centre should have access to all modalities of rehabilitation. This can be done by establishing strong links between the different lines of health care.

8.5 Components of pulmonary rehabilitation

8.5.1 Exercise training

As mentioned above, exercise training is now the cornerstone of rehabilitation, since it has a strong evidence base. A program of exercise training of the muscles of ambulation is recommended as a mandatory component of any pulmonary rehabilitation program. Exercise training should adhere to the general guidelines for exercise training in older adults. The goal of exercise training is to improve physical fitness. It should be distinguished from the goal of enhancing physical activity, which is the maintenance of optimal health.

To optimize health, light to moderate intense activities are advised in COPD, whereas physiological training effects occur at higher intensity. Strength training should also be advised in patients with respiratory disease, and flexibility training is advised to maintain joint range of motion. This has not been investigated specifically in patients with COPD, but there is no reason why stretching should not be applied. One study showed in a sham-controlled cross-over design improved shoulder mobility and discrete improvements of vital capacity after stretching of the pectoral muscle. Since patients with COPD have a 50% increased risk of falling and often suffer from severe osteoporosis which increases the risk of fractures, specific interventions to prevent falling may be advised in selected patients. When hospitalized with a hip fracture, patients suffering from COPD have 60 to 70% higher mortality compared to those without COPD.

8.5.1.1 *Whole-body exercise*

Exercise training has been included in virtually all studies investigating the benefits of pulmonary rehabilitation. In order to successfully increase skeletal muscle properties and render measurable physiological benefits, it is important that patients do exercise at relative high work loads. In COPD patients with primarily moderate disease, exercise training conducted at 75% of the peak work rate (60% of the difference between the lactate threshold and peak oxygen uptake) resulted in significant physiological effects. A similar training strategy was shown to be effective in patients with severe disease. Others have confirmed that high training intensity is required to elicit physiologic training effects.

Training load should be adapted in every training session, taking into account the patient's progression but also diurnal variability in the health condition of a patient. Trained staff should be available to

Table 8.2 Modifications that can be made to conventional whole-body endurance training to cope with ventilatory limitations of COPD patients

- Reduction of the time of exercise
  - Interval exercise training.
- Reduction of the ventilation to exercise or alleviating the work of breathing
  - Supplemental oxygen.
  - Non-invasive mechanical ventilation.
- Reduction simply of the amount of muscles put to work.
  - Single leg cycling.

ensure close supervision on the training intensity. Training intensity can be monitored using 10-point Borg symptom scales. A score around 4–6 is generally advised as an appropriate training intensity, provided the patients are familiar with the scale. As patients improve during training, the same Borg rating will be achieved at higher absolute work rates.

In patients who reach a ventilatory limitation during exercise, it is difficult to obtain a high training intensity for sustained periods of time due to dynamic hyperinflation and hypercapnia. Several strategies have been developed to ensure high-intensity training in more severe COPD (Table 8.2).

Obviously, in patients with COPD, optimal bronchodilatation is of utmost importance to ensure maximal training effects. A last intervention which enhances peak ventilatory capacity is bracing the arms. During walking this can be applied using a wheeled walking aid (rollator). Our group showed that bracing the arms on a rollator enhanced maximal voluntary ventilation by 8L/min, which partly explained the acute beneficial effect of a rollator. During treadmill walking, bracing of the arms can also easily be achieved.

8.5.1.2 *Resistance training*

Improving skeletal muscle function is an important goal of exercise training. Resistance training clearly specifically tackles the skeletal muscle. This form of exercise training, generally consisting of weight lifting, can be used as the only form of training, or in combination with whole-body exercises. In all the latter studies, muscle strength was significantly more increased when resistance training was added to the exercise regimen. Increased muscle strength is an important treatment objective in patients with COPD suffering from muscle weakness, as activities of daily life do require strength on top of muscle endurance. Patients suffering from muscle weakness may be particularly good candidates for a resistance training program.

Resistance training is easy to apply in clinical practice, and guidelines exist to build up strength training. The weight imposed and the number of repetitions ensure overload of the skeletal muscle. In patients with

COPD and several other chronic diseases resistance training is started at approximately 70% of the weight a patient can lift once (i.e. the 1 repetition maximum). The training volume (i.e. the number of repetitions times the resistance) can be increased by 2.5 to 5% per week. In male hypogonadal patients testosterone replacement therapy may enhance the gain in muscle strength after resistance training. Weekly intramuscular injections with testosterone, aiming at restoring testosterone levels to normal values in initially hypogonadal men, did enhance skeletal muscle force more than either of the interventions alone. Further studies are required to investigate the long-term safety of this intervention. However, since skeletal muscle dysfunction is in itself a negative prognostic factor, short-term use of testosterone may be beneficial to result in a rapid restoration of this potentially harmful situation.

8.5.1.3 *Neuromuscular electrical stimulation (NMES)*

This has been used to stimulate skeletal muscles in patients with COPD. Four studies have investigated successfully the effects of this intervention. Studies showed that there was more strength gain in the skeletal muscles treated with electrical stimulation, both as mono-therapy or in combination with general exercise training. This intervention may prove to be attractive in patients who have difficulties in taking part in regular rehabilitation, such as patients admitted to hospital with acute exacerbations.

8.5.1.4 *Inspiratory muscle training*

Specific training of the inspiratory muscles by threshold or resistive breathing or by isocapnic hyperpnea can be used in patients suffering from significant respiratory muscle weakness. This intervention alleviated dyspnoea and may—in selected patients—contribute to enhanced exercise performance. Inspiratory muscle training should be performed using sufficient inspiratory muscle load. With resistive or breathing or threshold loading at least 40% of the PImax should be generated.

8.5.2 Psychological counselling

In depressed patients (some 40% [95% CI: 36–44%] of patients with COPD), for example, *psychological counselling* may be of benefit in order to help reduce symptoms of depression or anxiety. Admittedly a large trial to confirm the point is currently still missing, but since depressive symptoms do significantly impact on health-related quality of life and even readmission in these patients, psychological counselling may well be worth the effort in patients who suffer from symptoms of depression, anxiety, or poor coping. It should be stressed, however, that exposure to exercise therapy may in itself have an antidepressant effect.

8.5.3 Nutritional interventions

Nutritional interventions have been shown to be unsuccessful in poorly selected COPD patients. However, when nutritional interventions are successful in improving body mass in cachectic patients, they do spin off in an important survival benefit. Besides patients suffering from pulmonary cachectia, a less recognized role, but likely of equal importance, is the care for obese COPD patients. Clearly obesity is linked to increased pulmonary ventilation to carry out activities of daily living. Consequently, weight loss, may, in obese patients, yield important functional benefits in activities carried out against gravity (e.g. stair climbing, walking). The authors believe that weight loss, particularly loss of fat mass, may be an important target in overweight COPD patients referred to pulmonary rehabilitation programs.

8.5.4 Occupational therapy

Occupational therapists may be consulted within the context of a rehabilitation program, and they may advise patients on the mode and pace of carrying out activities of daily life. Frequently, occupational therapists may advise on the use of wheeled walking aids (rollators). Although many patients show poor compliance with the daily use of a rollator, those who use it may substantially and suddenly improve their exercise tolerance.

8.5.5 Self-management

Other potentially cost-effective components of a rehabilitation program are interventions aiming at enhancing self-management. *Generally these interventions are supervised by specially trained advanced practice nurses*, who work integrated in the rehabilitation team. Interventions aiming at enhancing self-management have shown variable success. Studies showing cost-effectiveness of these interventions focussed on a subgroup of patients with at least one hospital admission. Hence it seems reasonable to direct efforts specifically to this subgroup of patients.

8.6 Maximizing long-term effectiveness of pulmonary rehabilitation: enhancing physical activity

In many studies the effects of pulmonary rehabilitation wear off relatively quickly. One of the reasons for this may be that pulmonary rehabilitation has not been always successful in achieving a more physically active life style. A minimum of 30min of physical activity of moderate intensity is critical to maintain health. A recent study showed the importance of maintaining a healthy and physically active life style to increase survival in COPD.

Only a handful of studies have investigated the effect of pulmonary rehabilitation on physical activity, and none of these studies were randomized controlled trials. Not all of them showed significant improvements of the amount and intensity of physical activities in daily life after pulmonary rehabilitation. One trial suggests that the effect of rehabilitation on physical activity is larger after longer programs. However, the relation between the length of the programs and their effectiveness on physical activity can surely not be seen across the different published trials.

The amount and intensity of activities in which patients engage depends, besides their exercise capacity, on intrinsic factors such as motivation, perceived self-efficacy, mood status, and health beliefs. Other factors related to physical activity are extrinsic factors such as social and cultural role, external barriers (e.g. environmental), and climate.

The missing link towards more endurable effects of pulmonary rehabilitation may very well be the failure to successfully enhance daily physical activity levels of patients sufficient to maintain health.

8.7 Conclusion

- Pulmonary rehabilitation is an evidence-based therapy for patients with COPD who have remaining symptoms of exercise intolerance and poor health-related quality of life, despite optimal medical therapy
- Patients who recently suffered from an acute exacerbation are good candidates for such programs
- Programs should be individually tailored in terms of the content and the format of the exercise training, the other disciplines involved in the setting of the program
- Particular attention should be given to ensure that patients become more physically active after pulmonary rehabilitation, since this may be the key to long-lasting effects of rehabilitation.

References

American College of Sports Medicine Position Stand (1998a). Exercise and physical activity for older adults. *Medicine and Science in Sports and Exercise*, **30**, 992–1008.

American College of Sports Medicine Position Stand (1998b). The recommended quantity and quality of exercise for developing and maintaining cardiorespiratory and muscular fitness, and flexibility in healthy adults. *Medicine and Science in Sports and* Exercise, **30**, 975–91.

Decramer M, Gosselink R, Troosters T, Verschueren M, and Evers G (1997). Muscle weakness is related to utilization of health care resources in COPD patients. *The European Respiratory Journal*, **10**, 417–23.

Haskell WL, Lee IM, Pate RR, *et al.* (2007). Physical activity and public health. Updated recommendation for adults from the American College of Sports Medicine and the American Heart Association. *Circulation*, **116**, 1081–93.

Lacasse Y, Goldstein R, Lasserson TJ, and Martin S (2006). Pulmonary rehabilitation for chronic obstructive pulmonary disease. *Cochrane Database of Systematic Reviews*, CD003793.

Lotters F, Van Tol B, Kwakkel G, and Gosselink R (2002). Effects of controlled inspiratory muscle training in patients with COPD: a meta-analysis. *The European Respiratory Journal*, **20**, 570–6.

Marquis K, Debigare R, Lacasse Y, *et al.* (2002). Midthigh muscle cross-sectional area is a better predictor of mortality than body mass index in patients with chronic obstructive pulmonary disease. *American Journal of Respiratory and Critical Care Medicine*, **166**, 809–13.

Nici L, Donner C, Wouters E, *et al.* (2006). American Thoracic Society/European Respiratory Society statement on pulmonary rehabilitation. *American Journal of Respiratory and Critical Care Medicine*, **173**, 1390–1413.

Pitta F, Troosters T, Probst V, Langer D, Decramer M, and Gosselink R (2008). Are patients with COPD more active after pulmonary rehabilitation. *Chest*, available online.

Puhan MA, Scharplatz M, Troosters T, and Steurer J (2005). Respiratory rehabilitation after acute exacerbation of COPD may reduce risk for readmission and mortality—a systematic review. *Respiratory Research*, **6**, 54.

Ries AL, Bauldoff GS, Carlin BW, *et al.* (2007). Pulmonary rehabilitation: Joint ACCP/AACVPR evidence-based clinical practice guidelines. *Chest*, **131** 4S–42S.

Troosters T, Casaburi R, Gosselink R, and Decramer M. (2005). Pulmonary rehabilitation in chronic obstructive pulmonary disease. *American Journal of Respiratory and Critical Care Medicine*, **172**, 19–38.

Chapter 9

Long-term, ambulatory, and short-burst oxygen therapy in COPD

Cassandra N.G. Lee and Onn Min Kon

Key points

- Long-term oxygen therapy (LTOT) has been demonstrated to improve survival in hypoxic chronic obstructive pulmonary disease (COPD) patients when used for >15 h a day.
- Criteria for LTOT are a pO_2 of <7.3kPa or pO_2 7.3–8kPa in patients with evidence of *cor pulmonale*.
- Ambulatory oxygen (AO) can improve desaturation and increase exercise capacity.
- Short-burst oxygen therapy (SBOT) may have a place in symptom relief.

9.1 Introduction

Long-term oxygen therapy (LTOT) improves survival in hypoxic patients with COPD. It has no or little effect on the decline in spirometry. The likely mechanism of the benefit of LTOT is by reducing the rate of worsening in pulmonary arterial hypertension in such patients. Chronic hypoxia is known to produce changes in the pulmonary vasculature with migration of smooth muscle cells into the intima and proliferation of these cells. There is subsequent remodelling of the vasculature with hypertrophy of the muscular media in the small pulmonary arteries, muscularization of the pulmonary arterioles and fibrosis of the intimal layer. Despite stabilizing the progression in pulmonary arterial hypertension, there is no evidence that LTOT reverses the non-cellular intimal fibrosis in post-mortem studies nor that it restores normal pulmonary arterial pressures.

9.2 Landmark studies of LTOT

9.2.1 The NOTT study 1980

In this unblinded study 203 patients with hypoxaemic COPD were randomized to either nocturnal oxygen therapy (n = 102) or continuous oxygen therapy (n = 101) at an oxygen flow rate of 1 to 4L/min. After 24 months of oxygen therapy, there was a significant improvement in mortality for the continuous oxygen therapy group (Figure 9.1). There were also significant decreases in the mean pulmonary artery pressure and pulmonary vascular resistance during exercise. In addition, continuous oxygen therapy was associated with larger decreases in resting and exercise pulmonary vascular resistance and significant improvements in the exercise response of mean pulmonary artery pressure and stroke index.

9.2.2 The MRC LTOT study 1981

Eighty-seven patients with a diagnosis of chronic bronchitis and emphysema were randomized to receive oxygen therapy or no oxygen. Patients were enrolled in the study if they had a PaO_2 of between 40 and 60mmHg (5.3 and 8kPa) and one or more recorded episodes of heart failure with ankle oedema. The treatment group received oxygen therapy for at least 15h a day. There was an improvement in mortality over 5yrs in the group receiving oxygen therapy.

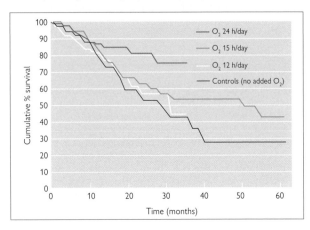

Figure 9.1 Survival in studies of long-term oxygen in COPD. The MRC study compared 15h with no oxygen, and the North American oxygen therapy trial compared 12h with attempted continuous oxygen.

Reproduced from the *BMJ* (1998), **317**: 871–4, with permission from the BMJ Publishing Group.

Currently there is no evidence to suggest that treating less severe patients with mild or moderate hypoxaemia results in any survival advantage. In addition, there is currently no evidence to suggest that treating patients with nocturnal desaturation/hypoxaemia alone improves survival.

9.3 **Practical guide to LTOT assessment and provision**

LTOT is the provision of oxygen therapy for continuous use at home for patients with chronic hypoxaemia (PaO_2 at or below 7.3kPa [55mHg]) (Table 9.1). This is normally delivered using an oxygen concentrator. The oxygen flow rate should be set to raise the oxygen tension above 8kPa (60mmHg). Once initiated, this therapy is likely to be life long. LTOT is given for at least 15h per day and includes the night time, given the presence of worsening arterial hypoxaemia during sleep.

An assessment should be made and it should demonstrate that the PaO_2 is consistently at or below 7.3kPa, when breathing air during a period of clinical stability (i.e. the absence of an exacerbation of the chronic lung disease for the previous five weeks). It should be stressed that the level of $PaCO_2$ does not influence the need for LTOT prescription. LTOT can also be prescribed in chronic hypoxia patients when the PaO_2 is between 7.3kPa and 8kPa, when there is the presence of polycythaemia or clinical and/or echocardiographic evidence of pulmonary hypertension.

Arterial blood gases (ABG's) from a radial or femoral artery or arterialized ear lobe capillary blood can be used for assessments. The patient should be breathing air for at least 30min after they last received any supplemental oxygen. ABGs should also be measured with the patient breathing supplemental oxygen for at least 30min to assess the change in the PaO_2 and $PaCO_2$.

It is usual to start with a supplemental oxygen flow rate of 2L/min via nasal cannulae, or from a 24% controlled oxygen face mask, and to aim for a PaO_2 value of at least 8kPa. If oxygenation is insufficient, the oxygen flow rate should be increased gradually. Some patients may require higher oxygen flow rates to correct hypoxaemia (greater than 4L/min) and thus may require an additional oxygen concentrator at home. There is no evidence of the benefit in increasing the oxygen flow rate routinely at night. In cases where there is excessive hypercapnia on attempting to adequately oxygenate the patient, chronic non-invasive ventilation may also be considered.

Smoking cessation techniques should be continued before any home oxygen assessment and prescription. Patients should be made

Table 9.1 Long-term oxygen therapy is generally indicated in severe COPD patients who have
• PaO_2 at or below 7.3kPa (55mmHg) or SaO_2 at or below 88%, with or without hypercapnia
or
• PaO_2 between 7.3kPa (55mmHg) and 8.0kPa (60mmHg), or SaO_2 of 88%, if there is evidence of pulmonary hypertension, peripheral oedema suggesting congestive cardiac failure, or polycythaemia (haematocrit >55%).

aware of the risks of continuing to smoke in the presence of home oxygen therapy, given the possibility of causing burns through the setting alight of the oxygen supply.

9.4 Ambulatory oxygen (AO) therapy

AO therapy can improve exercise tolerance and reduce dyspnoea at sub-maximal workloads (Figure 9.2). It can assist in reducing minute ventilation and dynamic hyperinflation. In addition, it may increase exercise endurance in the exercise-induced hypoxaemic patient.

Currently there is no evidence that AO has any long-term benefits, and the short-term benefits are limited. It should therefore only be prescribed after an assessment to determine the usage, oxygen flow rate, and acceptability of a device by the patient.

Patients requiring AO fall into two categories: (1) those with chronic hypoxaemia who fulfil the criteria for LTOT and (2) those who do not have chronic hypoxaemia but who have exercised induced hypoxemia.

9.4.1 LTOT patients and ambulatory oxygen

LTOT patients with limited mobility may require ambulatory oxygen to leave the house. This group of patients will not normally require an exercise test to determine flow rate, but rather it should be pre-scribed at the same level as LTOT with the aim of assessment and follow-up to determine usage and acceptability. Active patients should perform an exercise test to determine the flow rate that is sufficient to maximize exercise tolerance, reduce dyspnoea, and abolish desaturation whilst ensuring tolerability of the device. The goal should be to maintain SaO_2 > 90%—however, this may not always be possible, particularly not without significantly reducing the duration of delivery and therefore negating the benefits of portable oxygen.

9.4.2 Exercise desaturation and ambulatory oxygen

It is generally accepted that a fall in saturation on exertion of 4% to below 90% is considered significant. The aim of an assessment is to first confirm significant exercise desaturation and then to identify

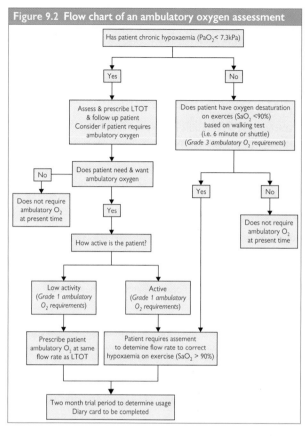

Figure 9.2 Flow chart of an ambulatory oxygen assessment

if supplemental oxygen can increase functional exercise tolerance or reduce dyspnoea, whilst abolishing/reducing desaturation, for the same given workload. The assessment is also used to determine the flow rate and ensure tolerability of the device. In this setting it is not necessary to compare performance with a placebo cylinder containing air.

Walking tests are likely to be the most sensitive exercise test to measure functional exercise tolerance. Both incremental and endurance, maximal, and sub-maximal tests can be used. However, the test should reflect the predicted level of exertion and purpose of use for AO. Assessments should be standardized with at least 30min recovery time between repeated exercise tests. All walking tests with oxygen should be performed on the same delivery system that the patient is going to use.

ABGs do not need to be routinely performed, but they may have a role in those patients with known CO_2 retention with increased FiO_2. Non-invasive SaO_2 monitors should be validated for ambulant use and be used throughout all exercise tests. For palliative care use, walking tests do not need to be performed; however, an assessment may be beneficial to determine the flow rate and suitability/tolerability of device.

9.4.3 Oxygen sources

These include concentrators and gas and liquid oxygen:

- Portable concentrators tend to be a pulsed delivery dose or, if constant, the flow rate is usually restricted to 4Lpm.
- Gas cylinders (Figure 9.3) can deliver a constant high flow rate, but duration is limited by cylinder size, which in turn directly impacts on weight and therefore portability. There are a variety of devices available that provide on-demand or pulsed dose delivery which can increase the duration of oxygen delivery by at least three- to four-fold fold and are generally well tolerated by patients.
- Liquid oxygen provides additional benefit and flexibility as it reduces the need for frequent deliveries—it is competitively lightweight and with comparatively good duration. However, it requires a certain level of dexterity and care when re-filling as serious freeze burns can occur.

Conserving devices function by targeting oxygen delivery with early inspiration, thereby increasing the duration of oxygen delivery source and can provide benefit for those patients with either high flow rates or who want to leave the house for prolonged periods. They are generally as effective as constant flow; however, patients should be assessed to determine the suitability. There is some evidence that they might not be as effective for mouth breathers or during maximal exercise.

Oxygen delivery devices are usually via dual pronged nasal cannulae (Figure 9.4); however, some patients may prefer a face mask or require a precise FiO_2. Few patients may benefit or require transtracheal oxygen; this should be performed by specialist teams and will require humidification, even at flow rates as low as 1Lpm.

Follow-up should be provided to establish subjective benefit and usage. To date there are no known predictors which identify patients that will use AO outside the house or to assist with activities of daily living. Diary records may be of benefit, and there is some evidence that AO may improve HRQoL (Health-related Quality of Life) outcome measures. AO should be withdrawn if unhelpful.

Figure 9.3 Ambulatory oxygen cylinder

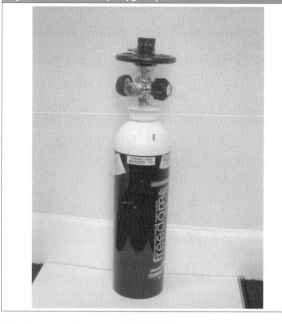

Figure 9.4 Patient using ambulatory oxygen

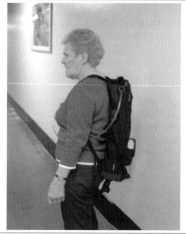

9.5 Short-burst oxygen therapy (SBOT)

SBOT refers to the intermittent use of oxygen, usually from a static cylinder. There is currently a lack of evidence to justify the routine use of SBOT, and once prescribed SBOT can be difficult to withdraw. For these reasons it is recommended that SBOT should only be started if there is objective evidence of benefit for the individual patient, and it should only be prescribed if an improvement in breathlessness and/or exercise tolerance can be documented.

No specific methodology has been developed for assessment for this mode of oxygen therapy; however, other causes of breathlessness must be excluded and patients should be assessed for LTOT if appropriate. In a selected group of patients with COPD there is some evidence that SBOT can shorten recovery time after activities of daily living. More research is required to identify those select patients who may have an objective benefit.

References

Bradley JM and O'Neill B (2005). Short term ambulatory oxygen for chronic obstructive pulmonary disease. *Cochrane Database of Systematic Reviews*, **4**, CD004356.

Bradley JM, Lasserson T, Elborn S, Macmahon J, and O'Neill B (2007). A systematic review of randomized controlled trials examining the short-term benefit of ambulatory oxygen in COPD. *Chest*, **131** (1), 278–85.

British Thoracic Society Working Group on Home Oxygen Services (2005). Clinical component on the assessment for provision of home oxygen services in England and Wales. *British Thoracic Society*.

Cranston JM, Crockett AJ, Moss JR, and Alpers JH (2005). Domiciliary oxygen for chronic obstructive pulmonary disease. *Cochrane Database of Systematic Reviews*, **4**, CD001744.

European Respiratory Society/American Thoracic Society (2004). Standards for the Diagnosis and Management of patients with COPD.

Fletcher EC, Luckett RA, Goodnight-White SA, Miller CC, Qian W, and Costarangos-Galarza C (1992). A double-blind trial of nocturnal supplemental oxygen for sleep desaturation in patients with chronic obstructive pulmonary disease and a daytime PaO_2 above 60mmHg. *American Review of Respiratory Disease*, **145** (5), 1070–6.

Górecka D, Gorzelak K, Sliwiński P, Tobiasz M, and Zieliński J (1997). Effect of long-term oxygen therapy on survival in patients with chronic obstructive pulmonary disease with moderate hypoxaemia. *Thorax*, **52** (8), 674–9.

Medical Research Council Working Party (1981). Long-term domiciliary oxygen therapy in chronic hypoxic *cor pulmonale* complicating chronic bronchitis and emphysema. *Lancet*, **i**, 681–6.

National Institutes of Health, National Heart, Lung and Blood Institute (Update 2006). Global strategy for the diagnosis, management, and prevention of chronic obstructive pulmonary disease. NHLBI/WHO Workshop Report.

NICE (2004). Managing stable COPD. *Thorax*, **59** (Suppl 1), i39–130.

Nocturnal Oxygen Therapy Trial Group (1980). Continuous or nocturnal oxygen therapy in hypoxemic chronic lung disease: a clinical trial. *Annals of Internal Medicine*, **93**, 391–8.

Nonoyama ML, Brooks D, Lacasse Y, Guyatt GH, and Goldstein RS (2007). Oxygen therapy during exercise training in chronic obstructive pulmonary disease. *Cochrane Database of Systematic Reviews*, **2**, CD005372.

Weitzenblum E, Sautegeau A, Ehrhart M, Mammosser M, and Pelletier A. (1985). Long-term oxygen therapy can reverse the progression of pulmonary hypertension in patients with chronic obstructive pulmonary disease. *American Review of Respiratory Disease*, **131** (4), 493–8.

Zieliński J, Tobiasz M, Hawryłkiewicz I, Sliwiński P, and Pałasiewicz G (1998). Effects of long-term oxygen therapy on pulmonary hemodynamics in COPD patients: a 6-year prospective study. *Chest,* **113** (1), 65–70.

Chapter 10

Lung volume reduction, bullectomy, and lung transplantation

William D. Man and Onn Min Kon

Key points

- Increased lung volumes are a characteristic of many patients with COPD and have negative mechanical effects on cardiopulmonary function.
- Lung volume can be reduced pharmacologically and surgically.
- The National Emphysema Treatment Trial (NETT) has identified selective subgroups that benefit from Lung Volume Reduction Surgery (LVRS) and has identified high-risk patients who should not be referred for LVRS.
- Less-invasive methods of lung volume reduction (bronchoscopic approach, airway bypass) are currently being evaluated.
- Bullectomy should be considered in breathless patients with a large bulla occupying greater than 30% of the hemithorax or a history of pneumothorax.

10.1 Introduction

Increased static and dynamic lung volumes are a characteristic of some patients with COPD, particularly those with severe disease. Emphysema is defined as the pathological enlargement of the airspaces distal to the terminal bronchiole, associated with destruction of the alveolar wall. Increased dynamic lung volumes arise from dynamic hyperinflation (DH), which results from expiratory flow limitation. As ventilation increases during exercise, lung emptying becomes incomplete, and hence lung volume fails to fall to its natural equilibrium point. Increased lung volumes have many negative mechanical effects, including the following:

- Altering the length-tension relationship of the respiratory muscles

- Increasing elastic load and work of breathing
- Limiting tidal volume expansion
- Impairing cardiac return and output.

Theoretically, interventions designed to reduce lung volumes in COPD patients should lead to improvements in cardiopulmonary mechanics with consequent improvements in symptoms and exercise capacity.

10.2 **Pharmacological lung volume reduction**

Bronchodilators are the mainstay of treatment in COPD. Despite minimal changes in forced expiratory volume in 1s (FEV_1), many patients describe symptomatic relief following bronchodilator therapy, principally through reductions in DH. Reductions in DH have been demonstrated in randomized controlled trials of short-acting and long-acting β_2-agonists and antimuscarinics. Helium and oxygen mixtures (*Heliox*) have also been shown to reduce breathlessness and improve exercise capacity in the laboratory exercise setting. Replacing nitrogen with helium reduces expiratory flow resistance and may improve lung emptying, thereby reducing DH. However, Heliox is yet to be used routinely in clinical practice.

10.3 **Lung volume reduction surgery (LVRS)**

LVRS was first proposed in the late 1950s when multiple wedge excisions were taken from the most affected portions of emphysematous lungs. However, there was high perioperative mortality (18%) and problems with persistent air leaks that prevented widespread uptake of the procedure. Improvements in surgical techniques and the introduction of materials to buttress the staple line have led to renewed interest recently, and several randomized controlled trials comparing LVRS with optimal medical treatment have now been published—the most important and largest being the National Emphysema Treatment Trial (NETT).

10.4 **The National Emphysema Treatment Trial (NETT)**

- *NETT* was a federally funded multi-centre, randomized controlled trial that recruited 1218 patients who had undergone pulmonary rehabilitation. Patients were randomized to LVRS or continued best medical therapy.
- An early statement was published highlighting excess mortality in high-risk patients (FEV_1 < 20% predicted and either diffusing

capacity for carbon monoxide (DLCO) < 20% predicted or homogenous emphysema on computed tomography [CT]. In 70 high-risk patients randomized to surgery, there was a 30-day mortality rate of 16% compared to no deaths in the 70 high-risk patients treated medically.

- In the non-high risk patients, LVRS, compared with medical therapy, increased mortality at 30 days (2.2% vs 0.2%) and at 90 days (5.2% vs 1.5%), but did not affect mortality at 2yrs. There appeared to be a small long-term survival benefit in favour of LVRS with a 5-yr risk ratio for death of 0.82.

- Sub-group analysis revealed that patients with predominantly *upper lobe emphysema* with *low exercise capacity* (<gender-specific 40% percentile) were most likely to benefit from LVRS. Five-year risk ratio for death was 0.57, and surgery was more likely to lead to short- and long-term improvement in exercise capacity (incremental cycle exercise) and health status (St.George's Respiratory Questionnaire).

- LVRS offered no survival benefit for patients with *upper lobe emphysema* and *high exercise capacity* but led to sustained improvements in exercise capacity and health status.

- Patients with predominantly *non-upper lobe emphysema* with *low exercise capacity* had no improved survival or exercise capacity with surgery but had limited improvement in health status that was not sustained at long-term follow-up.

- LVRS produced increased mortality at 90 days and 2 years, and made no improvements in exercise capacity or health status in patients with *non-upper lobe emphysema* and *high exercise capacity*.

- Figure 10.1 summarizes which patients should be referred for LVRS.

- No significant differences in either mortality or functional outcome have been found between median sternotomy technique and video assisted thoracoscopy (VAT) resection.

- Laser resection, when compared with stapled resection, have demonstrated lower improvements in FEV$_1$, increased mortality, higher costs, and increased length of hospital stay, and has therefore largely been abandoned.

10.5 **Bronchoscopic lung volume reduction**

Even in non-high risk patients, LVRS is not without risk, with significant morbidity, extended hospital stay, and an early mortality rate of 5%. Recent less-invasive approaches have included a bronchoscopic approach with *one-way valves* placed in airways leading to the most hyperinflated portions of the lung. The valve causes occlusion of the airway lumen, leading to lung collapse, but allows secretions to drain

Figure 10.1 Referral for LVRS

FEV$_1$ < 20% with either homogeneous emphysema or DLCO < 20% DO NOT REFER	
Upper lobe Emphysema Low Exercise Capacity REFER	Lower lobe Emphysema Low Exercise Capacity Consider referral only in very limited circumstances
Upper lobe Emphysema High Exercise Capacity Consider referral for symptomatic improvement	Lower lobe Emphysema High Exercise Capacity DO NOT REFER

and air to be emptied from the targeted lobe. Initial case series have shown promising results, although there have been concerns about risk of pneumothorax and limited efficacy due to extensive collateral ventilation. At the time of writing, the results of an international multi-centre randomized controlled study (the Endobronchial Valve for Emphysema Palliation Trial – VENT) are due to be published.

Other investigators have introduced biological agents to reduce lung volume by causing scarring of targeted lung areas, although human studies have only just commenced. Another bronchoscopic approach is the *airway bypass* technique that involves the insertion of stents between cartilaginous airways and emphysematous portions of the lung under endobronchial ultrasound guidance. This provides an additional low resistance pathway for expiration and reduction of gas trapping. There are promising pilot cases, and a randomized controlled trial is currently under way. This method may be particularly suitable for patients with homogeneous emphysema.

10.6 Bullectomy

A bulla is an air-filled, thin-walled space within the lung, which is greater than 1cm in diameter in the distended state. Bullous emphysema can cause substantial pulmonary dysfunction; removal of a bulla improves diaphragm configuration, increases elastic recoil pressure, improves dynamic compliance, and reduces airway resistance, functional residual capacity, and physiological dead space.

- The main indications for bullectomy are severe breathlessness in the setting of a large bulla occupying greater than 30% of the hemithorax or a history of pneumothorax.
- The benefits of bullectomy have been demonstrated by uncontrolled observational studies and case series, but not by a randomized controlled trial. In 60–90% of patients, there is significant improvement in terms of symptoms and lung function lasting several years.
- Perioperative mortality ranges from 0 to 10%. One report demonstrated 33% mortality in patients with significant cor pulmonale.

10.7 Lung transplantation

Unfortunately there are insufficient organs available to deal with the numbers of patients requiring transplantation. In addition to emphysema, worldwide major indications for lung transplantation comprise:

- Emphysema/COPD
- Cystic fibrosis
- Idiopathic pulmonary fibrosis
- Pulmonary hypertension
- Other diseases, for example, sarcoidosis, Langerhan's cell granulomatosis, lymphangioleiomyomatosis.

Referral for transplantation in COPD patients should only be considered in patients who continue to deteriorate despite maximal medical treatment, including smoking cessation, maximal bronchodilator treatment, pulmonary rehabilitation, and long-term oxygen therapy. In addition endoscopic or surgical lung volume reduction should also have been used where feasible. In addition to this lung transplantation patients with COPD only have a median survival of about 5yrs, with most failing secondary to obliterative bronchiolitis. Hence the appropriate timing for transplantation is complicated because extremely symptomatic COPD patients may have a relatively good prognosis and it is therefore sometimes finely balanced as to when this should be recommended.

Several factors should be considered when considering an individual's prognosis in relation to that following tranplantation:

- Hospitalization for an acute exacerbation associated with hypercapnia carries a 49% 2-year survival
- Survival rates decrease with increasing age, worsening hypoxemia, worsening hypercapnia, and increase in pulmonary artery pressure
- Survival rates decrease as FEV_1, DLCO, and BMI decrease.

- The BODE index may be a useful prognostic score—includes the BMI, the percent predicted FEV_1, the degree of dyspnoea and the exercise capacity (assessed by the 6-min walk distance). A BODE index of 7 to 10 (on a scale from 0 to 10) was associated with a median survival of about 3yrs. Patients with a score of 5 to 6 can be referred early prior to progression of disease.
- The NETT study identified a high-risk group of patients with a median survival of about 3yrs with medical therapy–patients with an FEV_1 of less than 20% and either a DLCO of less than 20% or homogeneously distributed emphysema.

10.8 Specific guidelines for transplantation in COPD (International Society for Heart and Lung Transplantation 2006)

Patients with a BODE index of 7 to 10 or at least 1 of the following:

   a) History of hospitalization for exacerbation associated with acute hypercapnia (pCO_2 exceeding 6.67kPa or 50mmHg)
   b) Pulmonary hypertension or *cor pulmonale*, or both, despite oxygen therapy.
   c) FEV_1 of less than 20% and either DLCO of less than 20% or homogenous distribution of emphysema.

10.9 Relative contraindications for lung transplantation

- Age >65 yrs
- Critical /unstable clinical condition (e.g. shock, mechanical ventilation)
- Severely limited functional status with poor rehabilitation potential
- Colonization with highly resistant or highly virulent bacteria, fungi, or mycobacteria
- Obesity (BMI >30kg/m^2)
- Severe osteoporosis
- Other medical conditions that have not led to end-stage organ damage need to be optimally treated before transplantation (e.g. diabetes).

Key references

Belman MJ, Botnick WC, and Shin JW (1996). Inhaled bronchodilators reduce dynamic hyperinflation during exercise in patients with chronic obstructive pulmonary disease. *American Journal of Respiratory and Critical Care Medicine,* **153** (3), 967–75.

Celli BR, Cote CG, Marin JM, et al. (2004). The body-mass index, airflow obstruction, dyspnea, and exercise capacity index in chronic obstructive pulmonary disease. *The New England Journal of Medicine,* **350** (10):1005–12.

Fishman A, Martinez F, Naunheim K, et al. (2003). A randomized trial comparing lung-volume-reduction surgery with medical therapy for severe emphysema. *The New England Journal of Medicine,* **348** (21), 2059–73.

Naunheim KS, Wood DE, Douglas E, et al. (2006). Long-term follow-up of patients receiving lung-volume-reduction surgery versus medical therapy for severe emphysema by the National Emphysema Treatment Trial Research Group. *The Annals of Thoracic Surgery,* **82** (2), 431–43.

Orens JB, Estenne M, Arcasoy S, et al. (2006). International Guidelines for the Selection of Lung Transplant Candidates: 2006 Update—A Consensus Report From the Pulmonary Scientific Council of the International Society for Heart and Lung Transplantation. *The Journal of Heart and Lung Transplantation,* **25** (7), 745–55.

Palange P, Valli G, Onorati P, et al. (2004). Effect of heliox on lung dynamic hyperinflation, dyspnea, and exercise endurance capacity in COPD patients. *Journal of Applied Physiology,* **97** (5), 1637–42.

Palla A, Desideri M, Rossi G, et al. (2005). Elective surgery for giant bullous emphysema: a 5-year clinical and functional follow-up. *Chest,* **128** (4), 2043–50.

Reilly J, Washko G, Pinto-Plata V, et al. (2007). Biological lung volume reduction: a new bronchoscopic therapy for advanced emphysema. *Chest,* **131** (4), 1108–13.

Toma TP, Hopkinson NS, Hillier J, et al. (2003). Bronchoscopic volume reduction with valve implants in patients with severe emphysema. *Lancet,* **361** (9361), 931–3.

Chapter 11

Palliative care and end-of-life issues

David J. Jackson and Sarah L. Elkin

> ### Key points
> - Palliative care needs of patients with advanced COPD remain unmet.
> - Despite difficulties predicting the precise prognosis in severe COPD—palliative care input should be considered at all stages.
> - Breathlessness can be treated with anxiolytics, opioids, and oxygen.
> - Palliative care involves the management of symptoms but also psychological, social, and spiritual problems.
> - Anxiety and depression are often overlooked and require treatment.

11.1 Introduction

The word 'palliate' comes from the Latin word 'palliare' meaning 'to cloak'. The Oxford English Dictionary defines palliate (in the context of health care) as alleviating symptoms of a disease without curing it. The World Health Organization defines palliative care as care that is patient and family centered, optimizing quality of life by anticipating, preventing, and treating suffering. It is most commonly associated with cancer, but the symptomatology of cancer and non-cancer patients is often similar, and whilst cancer patients' symptoms may be more severe, those of non-cancer patients tend to be more prolonged.

COPD is the commonest chronic respiratory disease requiring palliation. Palliative care throughout the continuum of illness involves addressing physical, intellectual, emotional, social, and spiritual needs (Figure 11.1), facilitating patient autonomy, access to information, and choice. 'End-of-life' care is one part of palliative care, the latter distinguished in part through its emphasis on maximizing quality of life prior to this final stage.

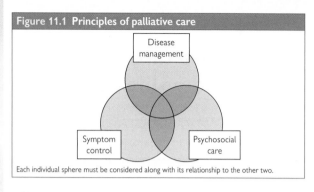

Understanding the natural history of disease allows the clinician to predict how long a person with an incurable disease might live for and the trajectory of their decline. In the case of malignant disease, although individual cancers behave differently, predictions of prognosis and life expectancy relate to grade and stage and are well described in the literature. The evolution of COPD particularly in the end stages differs from cancer with a trajectory that is characterized by frequent exacerbations and fluctuating symptoms (Figure 11.2). Patients with COPD often remain relatively stable, albeit at a low level, only to deteriorate acutely and unpredictably. Unfortunately, patients with advanced COPD often present to A+E in extremis, necessitating rushed decisions about intubation and ventilation with little information available about their previous quality of life or wishes about resuscitation.

11.2 Issues in palliative care

11.2.1 End-of-life decision making

The pattern of health decline in COPD patients does not fit the traditional hospice model well and may explain why patients dying from end-stage COPD are less likely to be offered hospice care when compared to those with cancer. Indeed health care for these patients is often initiated in response to acute exacerbations rather than proactively based on a previously developed management plan. Patients themselves may not be able to differentiate their final exacerbation from any other and fail to recognize it until their final hours. The 'SUPPORT' study prospectively looked at over 9000 adults with the primary objective of improving end-of-life decision making used APACHE II scores (a marker of deranged physiology) to create a prognostic model. This study showed that 5 days prior to death

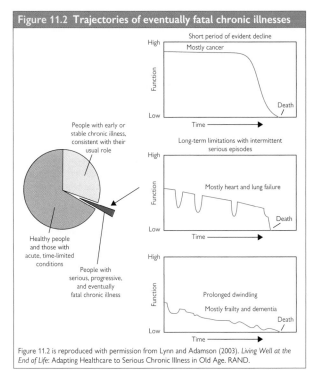

Figure 11.2 is reproduced with permission from Lynn and Adamson (2003). *Living Well at the End of Life*: Adapting Healthcare to Serious Chronic Illness in Old Age. RAND.

patients with lung cancer were predicted to have <10% chance of surviving 6 months, whereas those with COPD were predicted to have >50% chance. In other studies, just over half of the relatives of recently deceased patients with COPD were unaware that the deceased might die. Yet many of these patients were housebound with a high symptom burden and most were admitted at least twice in the year before death. The significant inability to predict death in these patients is at the heart of why so few receive adequate palliative care until the very last hours of life and, even less, the kind of passing that they desire. Research shows that despite the preference amongst the majority of COPD patients for treatment focused on comfort rather than on prolonging life, they frequently die in the ICU, having been mechanically ventilated with severe dyspnoea. The same is not true for those with lung cancer despite similar desires for intubation and cardiopulmonary recuscitation (CPR).

The uneven trajectory of decline in COPD patients has made it difficult to devise clear guidelines on when to refer to palliative care services. There is, however, a growing evidence base linking certain disease characteristics to earlier mortality. A scale consisting of body mass index (BMI), exercise capacity, and subjective estimates of dyspnoea has been shown to help predict survival over 1–3 years (Celli 2004). Other poor prognostic indicators are increasing age, recurrent hospital admission, poor functional status, depression, co-morbid illnesses, forced expiratory volume in 1s (FEV$_1$) <35% predicted, poor quality of life and low PaO$_2$. It has been suggested that criteria for hospice admission should include factors such as *cor pulmonale*, low albumin, weight loss >10%, low PaO$_2$ despite oxygen therapy and poor functional status (Fox *et al.* 1999).

If referring to palliative care services it is important the patient is in agreement and there are symptoms or issues requiring their expert input. A rough prognosis is often required by the accepting teams.

11.2.2 Advanced directives

Over the past decade a growing body of evidence highlights a considerable lack of communication regarding end-of-life issues in COPD despite a similar disease burden to cancer. This is in spite of a shift in attitudes in recent years towards complete disclosure of information to patients. The current literature highlights that only a third of oxygen-dependent patients with COPD have an end-of-life discussion with their doctor. Studies have demonstrated that patients wish to be informed of:

- The disease process, treatment, and prognosis
- What their death might be like
- Advanced care planning
- Emotional support
- Health care professionals who are accessible (Curtis *et al.*, 2004).

Many health care professionals believe that introducing the topic of terminal care will cause unnecessary stress and upset both the patient and their family and that the information conflicts with their need to protect the patient and retain an optimistic outlook. Moreover, some feel that they lack the confidence in communicating at the end of life and are unsure about what care is available for the patient. As there is frequently uncertainty with regard to prognosis there is further difficulty in both how and when to discuss end-of-life issues. Although estimating prognosis is an inexact science, prognostic uncertainty should not prevent us from talking with our patients as a number will die suddenly and we will have done them a disservice if end-of-life issues have not been addressed.

Evidence suggests that patients can engage in such discussions with minimal stress and that most patients prefer to discuss these issues relatively early on in the course of their disease when the stresses are less. There is further evidence illustrating that avoidance can lead to poorer patient satisfaction accompanied by feelings of anxiety and higher levels of depression.

Health care professionals do, however, need to be sensitive to those patients who prefer to turn a blind eye to the full reality of their condition. Coping mechanisms and desire for knowledge about prognosis vary greatly from patient to patient, and it must be appreciated that different individuals require different information.

11.2.3 Health care needs

Knowledge of health care needs in end-stage COPD is still developing and there are few definitions of a desirable standard of care.

Studies have revealed that patients wish to have more help to meet their physical and wider needs earlier in the disease and more help dealing with symptoms of breathlessness, depression, and fear. It appears that patients get more help with physical complaints rather than emotional issues. There also appears to be a lack of social support and prognostic information. Lastly, many patients die in hospital without the possibility or choice of dying at home.

Often in today's NHS the patient will be known to a 'COPD team' and will have formed a relationship with someone within that team. These specialist care workers are able to offer excellent supportive care as regards emotional support, education, and day-to-day symptom control but are less skilled at advanced care planning and end stage/terminal care.

Palliative care workers are used to dealing with advanced care planning and are highly skilled at delivering end-of-life care but often admit they need upskilling in COPD. A logical approach, therefore, appears to be a joint approach, perhaps with introduction to the palliative care team earlier in the disease process, some joint visits, and a dip-in/dip-out service from palliative care as necessary with more intensive expert input at the end of life. This approach will also enable upskilling of both parties.

Many UK hospices would need increased financial resource to increase capacity to care for patients with COPD. There is some emerging evidence that improving palliative care services for patients with COPD would lead to a decrease in hospital admissions and inappropriate, unwanted ITU stays and thus reduce cost. The end-of-life strategy and palliative care NSF would support expansion of current service/staffing levels.

11.3 Symptoms and clinical issues

The main symptoms reported by patients with end-stage COPD are discussed below.

11.3.1 Breathlessness

It is important to appreciate the impact of dyspnoea on the patient. Many are terrified by the thought of dying during an episode of acute breathlessness and have fears of suffocation. No patient should die with distressing breathlessness, and failure to relieve terminal breathlessness is a failure to utilize drug treatment correctly. Regular nebulized bronchodilators provide only modest relief for these patients, and it is important to be aware of alternative therapies.

11.3.2 Depression and anxiety

In many diseases there is a recognized reluctance of doctors to diagnose and treat mental health problems in those with physical illness. There is the view that 'reactive' psychological morbidity is an inevitable consequence of chronic physical disease and is refractory to treatment.

The majority of patients with COPD are smokers or ex-smokers, and many feel their disease is self-inflicted. The stress and anxiety they feel about this is inevitably mirrored by their relatives and carers. They are often housebound and attached to oxygen for the majority of the day. Walking 10 steps to the toilet can mean a 15-min recovery period as they struggle to get their breath back. It is not difficult to perceive how easy it is for them to become depressed at the hopelessness and helplessness of their situation. In fact, there is evidence that both the prevalence and severity of anxiety and depression amongst those with end-stage COPD is greater than in those with non-small cell lung cancer.

Many of the biological symptoms of depression such as fatigue, sleep disturbance, and weight loss are common in advanced COPD, and this in part explains the finding that less than half of those with severe depression or anxiety are being treated. One of the consequences of depression is that it can alter the patients' ability to fully understand the impact of the decisions that they make, and there is evidence that not only do these patients have a stronger preference for 'Do Not Attempt Resuscitation' (DNAR) orders but that their treatment preferences change after the depression resolves. Furthermore, there is some evidence that antidepressants not only improve mood but can also improve the subjective feeling of dyspnoea. The importance of recognizing and treating depression is further supported by the recent study that links depression to earlier mortality and longer inpatient stays in COPD.

11.3.3 Weight loss

Many patients with end-stage COPD have a low body mass index and are nutritionally deplete. They appear to have an increased resting energy expenditure linked to systemic inflammation with an accelerated loss of skeletal muscle. This cachexia is often poorly responsive to nutritional interventions. It appears that semi-starvation and muscle atrophy are equally distributed among disease stages, but the highest prevalence of cachexia is reported in Global Initiative for Chronic Obstructive Lung Disease (GOLD) Stage IV (Ambrosino and Simmonds 2007).

Several studies have found higher mortality rates in underweight individuals. Poor nutritional status is an independent risk factor for mortality and hospitalization in those receiving Long-term oxygen therapy (LTOT).

11.3.4 **Fatigue**

Fatigue is a common symptom in patients with severe COPD and can have a profound effect on their quality of life. It is important to rule out any contributing factors such as anaemia or depression and to review their medication.

Advice on breathing control and pacing activities as well as an explanation on why they feel so tired can help reassure the patient. Attention to nutritional intake is also important.

11.3.5 **Noisy, moist breathing (death rattle)**

In the final hours of life secretions can build up in the hypopharynx, oscillating in time with inspiration and expiration to produce a rattling noise. This is usually most distressing for relatives, carers, and other patients nearby rather than the patient themselves who frequently has a reduced conscious level secondary to hypercapnia and/or drug effects. Explaining to the family that their relative is not distressed by the rattle will greatly ease their anxiety. Positioning the patient in a semi-prone position encourages postural drainage, and, if needed, an antimuscarinic drug such as glycopyrronium or hyoscine can be used. Hyoscine in addition possesses sedative and anti-emetic properties as it crosses the blood brain barrier, and this may be useful if there is nausea due to opioids.

11.4 **Treatment Options**

As the severity of disease increases, therapy aimed to prolong life become less important in comparison to palliative therapy aimed to relieve symptoms. The evidence base for symptom control in end-stage COPD is lacking, and management relies on a mix of extrapolated evidence and personal experience.

11.4.1 **Opioids**

Opiates decrease ventilatory demand by decreasing the central drive. The concern with opioids in any chest patient is the fear of worsening respiratory failure. A trial of opioids in patients without hypercapnia is appropriate with close monitoring. However, in the terminal phase, opioid therapy is completely justified even in the presence of type 2 respiratory failure if the dyspnoea is severe. Low doses and small increments should be used (e.g. 2.5–5mg morphine p.o prn or 4-hourly). Opioids are also excellent antitussives.

Although lacking an evidence base, other non-pharmacological means of reducing dyspnoea include cool air from a fan or open window, massage, aromatherapy, positioning, and other relaxation methods.

11.4.2 **Anxiolytics**

There is little doubt that anxiety can exacerbate breathlessness and hospital admission, and clinical experience supports a role for a low-dose benzodiazepine despite a paucity of evidence in the literature. Lorazepam 1–2mg works fast but has a shorter half-life than diazepam, and there is therefore a risk of reactive agitation as the effect wears off. If, however, it is prescribed in the evening the patient can fall asleep in a more settled and comfortable state without the grogginess in the morning. Owing to its long half-life, the alternative benzodiazepine diazepam will accumulate even at low doses, and it therefore needs to be used with caution. In some patients (unlicensed use in the absence of depression) an *SSRI* may be helpful, either alone or in combination with a benzodiazepine.

11.4.3 **Oxygen therapy**

LTOT has been shown to reduce all-cause mortality in patients with resting hypoxaemia (aterial O_2 tension <8Kpa). Although clinicians feel positive when prescribing oxygen to COPD patients they should realize this is a huge milestone for many patients who recognize they are deteriorating and often feel negative about the transition. This might be a useful point to offer more support to the patient and carers.

The level of hypoxia does not necessarily correlate with the degree of dyspnoea in end-stage disease, and whilst most patients meet criteria for continuous oxygen at home others do not. In this latter group of patients, relief of dyspnoea through short-burst oxygen therapy might be gained, although this may simply be through a reduction in anxiety or the effect of facial or nasal cooling.

It should be noted that in a 6-month trial of short-burst O_2 treatment in patients with severe COPD there was no significant difference in either the health status of the patients or the healthcare utilization when they had access to as-needed O_2 therapy (Eaton 2006). Interestingly, the number of cylinders used during the study declined steadily, suggesting an early placebo effect.

Lastly, the evidence for ambulatory oxygen as a way of improving exercise performance is good, and this should be offered to appropriate patients alongside careful assessment.

11.5 Conclusion

The nature of COPD is such that the final time period will vary from days to months depending on the trajectory of the individual patients' illness. In the last year of life patients with COPD have a heavy symptom load. They have physical symptoms typical of COPD, such as breathlessness as well as other symptoms of depression, anxiety, and pain. The need for a palliative care approach involving not only control of symptoms but management of psychological, social, and spiritual problems is apparent in everyday clinical practice and is supported by the literature. Currently the palliative care needs of patients with advanced COPD remain unmet and in reality are no less necessary than in the context of lung cancer. The responsibility to educate patients with severe COPD about end-of-life care rests with the physicians caring for them. They must ensure that psychological problems are recognized and that their patients receive the care they desire most at the end of their life. A multidisciplinary approach involving physiotherapists, occupational therapists, palliative care specialists, as well as respiratory nurses and physicians is the only way this can fully be achieved.

The National Council of Palliative Care state in their website 'Our continuing mission is to ensure that all those suffering from life-threatening conditions, who need palliative care, receive it.' Let us hope this vision is realized for our severe patients with COPD.

References

Albert P and Calverley PM (2008). Drugs (including oxygen) in severe COPD. *The European Respiratory Journal*, **31** (5), 1114–24.

Ambrosino N and Goldstein R (2007). Series on comprehensive management of end-stage COPD. *The European Respiratory Journal*, **30** (5), 828–30.

Ambrosino N and Simmonds A (2007). The clinical management in extremely severe COPD. *Respiratory Medicine*, **101** (8), 1613–24.

Au DH, Udris EM, Fihn SD, McDonell MB, and Curtis JR (2006). Differences in health care utilisation at the end of life among patients with COPD and patients with lung cancer. *Archives of Internal Medicine*, **166** (3), 326–31.

Borson S, McDonald GJ, Gayle T, *et al*. (1992). Improvement in mood, physical symptoms, and function with nortrptyline for depression in patients with COPD. *Psychosomatics*, **33**, 190–201.

Celli BR, Cote CG, Marin JM, *et al*. (2004). The body mass index, airflow obstruction, dyspnoea and exercise capacity index in COPD. *The New England Journal of Medicine*, **350** (10),1005–12.

Claessens MT, Lynn J, Zhong Z, *et al*. (2000). Dying with lung cancer or COPD: insights from SUPPORT. *Journal of the American Geriatrics Society*, **48** (Suppl 5), S146–53.

Clayton JM, Hancock KM, Butow PN, *et al*. (2007).Clinical practice guidelines for communicating prognosis and end-of-life issues with adults in the advanced stages of a life-limiting illness, and their caregivers. *The Medical Journal of Australia*, **186** (Suppl 12), S77–108.

Connors AFJ, Dawson NV, Thomas C, et al. (1996). Outcomes following acute exacerbation of severe chronic obstructive lung disease. The SUPPORT investigators (Study to Understand Prognoses and Preferences for Outcomes and Risks of Treatments). *American Journal of Respiratory and Critical Care Medicine*, **154**, 959–67.

Curtis JR, Cook DJ, Sinuff T, et al. (2007). Noninvasive positive pressure ventilation in critical and palliative care settings: understanding the goals of therapy. *Critical Care Medicine*, **35**(3), 932–39.

Curtis JR, Wenrich MD, Carline JD, et al. (2001). Understanding physicians' skills at providing end-of-life care: perspectives of patients, families, and health care workers. *Journal of General Internal Medicine*, **16**, 41–9.

Gaber KA, Barnett M, Planchant Y, and McGavin CR (2004). Attitudes of 100 patients with COPD to artificial ventilation and cardiopulmonary resuscitation. *Palliative Medicine*, **18**, 626–9.

Curtis JR. Engelberg RA, Nielsen EL, et al. (2004). Patient-physician communication about end-of-life care for patients with severe COPD. *The European Respiratory Journal*, **24**, 200–5.

Elkington H, White P, Addington-Hall J, Higgs R, and Edmonds P (2005). The healthcare needs of COPD patients in the last year of life. *Palliative Medicine*, **19**, 485–91.

Fabbri LM, Luppi F, Beghe B, et al. (2008). Complex chronic comorbidities of COPD. *The European Respiratory Journal*, **31** (1), 204–12.

Fox E, Landrum-McNiff K, Zhong Z, Dawson NV, Wu AW, and Lynn J (1999). Evaluation of prognostic criteria for determining hospice eligibility in patients with advanced lung, heart or liver disease. *JAMA*, **282** (17), 1638–45.

Gore JM, Brophy CJ, and Greenstone MA (2000). How well do we care for patients with end stage COPD? A comparison of palliative care and quality of life in COPD and lung cancer. *Thorax*, **55**, 1000–6.

Heffner JE, Fahy B, Hilling L, et al. (1997). Outcomes of advance directive education of pulmonary rehabilitation patients. *American Journal of Respiratory and Critical Care Medicine*, **155**, 1055–9.

Hill K, Geist R, Goldstein RS, et al. (2008). Anxiety and depression in end-stage COPD. *The European Respiratory Journal*, **31** (3), 667–77.

Knauft ME, Nielsen EL, Engelberg RA, Patrick DL, and Curtis JR (2005). Barriers and facilitators to communication about end-of-life care for patients with severe COPD. *Chest*, **127** (2), 188–96.

Hansen-Flaschen J (2004). COPD: The last year of life. *Respiratory Care*, **49**(1), 90–7.

Kunik ME, Roundy K, Veazey C, et al. (2005). Surprisingly high prevalence of anxiety and depression in chronic breathing disorders. *Chest* **127**, (4), 1205–11.

Rosenfeld KE, Wenger NS, Phillips RS, et al. (1996). Factors associated with change in resuscitation preferences of seriously ill patients. *Archives of Internal Medicine*, **156**, 1558–64.

Index

111